THE POCKET GUIDE TO PHYSIOLOGIC ARTERIAL TESTING

For Peripheral Artery Disease

ROBERT J. DAIGLE, JR. BA, RVT, FSVU, FSDMS

Published by Summer Publishing

Printed November 2013, August 2014, November 2014
Rev.1

Summer Publishing, LLC.
4572 Christensen Circle
Littleton, CO 80123

303-734-1789
fax- 1-866-519-0674
email address: Sales@SummerPublishing.com
website: www.summerpublishing.com

Book illustrations by Rodney Summer
Cover design by Pam McKinnie, Concepts Unlimited

ISBN 978-0-9899329-0-5

INTRODUCTION

Peripheral arterial disease (PAD) affects 8-12 million Americans.[1] Some estimate that 20% of those over 70 years of age have PAD. About 1 in 3 people older than 50 who has diabetes also has PAD.[2] Unfortunately, the condition goes undetected in many patients.

An abnormal ankle to brachial index (ABI), in addition indicating the presence of PAD, is also a "marker" for coronary heart disease. A patient with an abnormal ABI has 3 to 4 fold increase in risk for cardiovascular death.[3]

Noninvasive physiologic arterial testing is a low-cost, efficient method of detecting arterial disease in the lower and upper extremities. Additionally, it can provide a method for identifying patients that are at high risk for stroke and myocardial infarct (MI).

This pocket guide will provide the following information:

⇒ Essential lessons in arterial hemodynamics and anatomy.

⇒ Diagnostic instrumentation is explained in theory and practical applications are demonstrated.

⇒ The recommended methods will follow recent changes to CMS-Medicare local coverage determination policy, and the consensus recommendations for ABI methods from the American Heart Association.[4]

⇒ Specific testing protocols are defined and step-by-step instructions are given.

⇒ Case studies are provided with a discussion of each case.

⇒ Common pitfalls in methods and interpretation are illustrated.

⇒ Instruction for diagnosing upper extremity arterial diseases.

⇒ Reimbursement information and guidelines.

This book will not instruct diagnostic methods using Color Duplex Ultrasound. Noninvasive physiologic testing should be the primary test method, and duplex ultrasound used (optionally) if the physiologic study is abnormal. For information of Color Duplex imaging of native vessels, stents and bypass grafts, consult Techniques in Noninvasive Vascular Diagnosis from Summer Publishing (www.Summerpublishing.com)

References

1. Vascular Disease Foundation. www.vdf.org
2. NIH- http://www.nhlbi.nih.gov/health/health-topics/topics/pad/atrisk.html
3. Hiatt WR, Nehle MR. Peripheral Arterial Disease. American Medical Network. http://www.health.am/vein/peripheral-arterial-disease
4. Aboyans V, et. al. Measurement and Interpretation of the Ankle-Brachial Index. A Scientific Statement From the American Heart Association. Circulation. 2012;126:00-00.

TABLE OF CONTENTS

CHAPTER 1: ANATOMY & HEMODYNAMICS

ATHEROSCLEROSIS

Atherosclerosis is a condition in which an artery wall thickens as a result of the accumulation of fatty materials such as cholesterol and triglyceride. The condition involves a chronic inflammatory response in the walls of arteries caused largely by the accumulation of macrophages and white blood cells, and promoted by low-density lipoproteins (LDL). It is commonly referred to as "hardening of the arteries". Multiple athero plaques that form within the arteries can narrow or occlude the lumen.[1]

Risk Factors

* familial-generic component
* cholesteral >240 mg/dl
* hypertension
* diabetes mellitus
* severe obesity
* elevated triglycerides
* hypercholesterolemia
* LDL > 160 mg/dl
* tobacco abuse
* depressed fibrinolytic system
* increased oxidation of LDLs

SYMPTOMS OF PERIPHERAL ARTERIAL DISEASE (PAD)

With the exception of thromboemboli, arterial symptoms are chronic and take a long time to develop.

Mild arterial disease:

- Asymptomatic.
- May have decreased pedal pulses, or arterial bruit.
- With exercise, a slight decrease in ankle pressure.
- No significant reduction in blood flow at rest.

Moderate disease:

- Asymptomatic at rest.

- With exercise, a significant decrease in ankle pressure.
- Intermittent claudication is the most common symptom of PAD: pain, fatigue or cramping in the calf, thigh or buttock with exercise. Symptoms are relieved by rest. Claudication is brought about by a transient ischemic condition in the muscles.

Severe disease:

- Night pain - ischemic pain that occurs in the feet or toes at night when the patient is supine. It is relieved by sitting up or standing (leg dependent).
- Ischemic rest pain in feet and toes (persistent).
- Non-healing wounds on feet/toes.
- Ulceration on lower leg or feet.
- Tissue necrosis, gangrene in the feet/toes.
- Severe PAD requires surgical intervention to revascularize the limb. Alternatively, limb amputation is required.
- The five P's (pain, pallor, pulselessness, paresthesias, and paralysis) are a sign of acute obstruction.

Symptoms NOT Associated with Arterial Disease

These symptoms are more likely to be associated with venous disease or some other condition:

⇒ Acute onset, persistent pain in the calf or thigh.

⇒ Limb swelling and limb warmth.

⇒ Limb cyanosis.

⇒ Local tenderness.

Arterial Pathologies

⇒ Atherosclerosis. This is the primary circulatory disease affecting the lower extremities. If the disease is present, the predominate location for severe narrowing or occlusion is in the distal femoral artery. Diabetic patients have a propensity to develop athero disease in the tibial vessels.

⇒ Thrombosis. (spontaneous arterial thrombosis is uncommon, unless severe flow-restrictive lesions are present).

⇒ Thromboemboli (often originating from aneurysms). If emboli are small, they may occlude small vessels in the feet or toes. If large, they may obstruct major arteries. Symptoms are acute in onset.

⇒ "Blue toe" syndrome. Acute onset, painful cyanotic regions on toes or foot, caused by thromboemboli; also known as "trash foot".

⇒ Buerger's disease (aka, thromboangiitis obliterans). Small vessel "fixed" occlusive disease, most often occurring in the digits of male smokers.

⇒ Digit vasospastic disorder. Raynaud's Syndrome, episodic, prolonged digital vasospasm.

⇒ Aneurysm. A dilation and expansion of the arterial walls. The lumen may contain thrombus

⇒ Pseudoaneurysms. Not associated with atherosclerosis. A high-pressure extravasation of blood flow into the surrounding tissue.

⇒ Arteritis, giant cell arteritis. An inflammatory process of the arterial wall affecting medium and large arteries.

⇒ Entrapment syndromes. Arterial flow that is restricted by structures that extrinsically pinch or constrict an artery.

- Popliteal artery entrapment - claudication symptoms in the calf due to intermittent compression of the popliteal artery.
- Thoracic outlet syndrome - intermittent, positional compression of the subclavian or axillary artery.
- Nutcracker syndrome - renal vein entrapment.
- Median arcuate syndrome - compression of the celiac axis. Also, SMA syndrome - compression of the superior mesenteric artery.

ARTERIAL ANATOMY OF THE LOWER EXTREMITIES

- Abdominal Aorta (AA) - branches into 2 common iliac arteries at the level of the umbilicus (belly-button).
- Common Iliac artery (CIA) - branches into the internal iliac and external iliac arteries in the pelvis.
- Internal iliac a. (IIA) (also known as the hypogastric artery) - supplies blood flow to the pelvis, buttock area, and reproductive organs.
- External iliac a. (EIA) - becomes the common femoral artery at the inguinal ligament (at the groin crease).

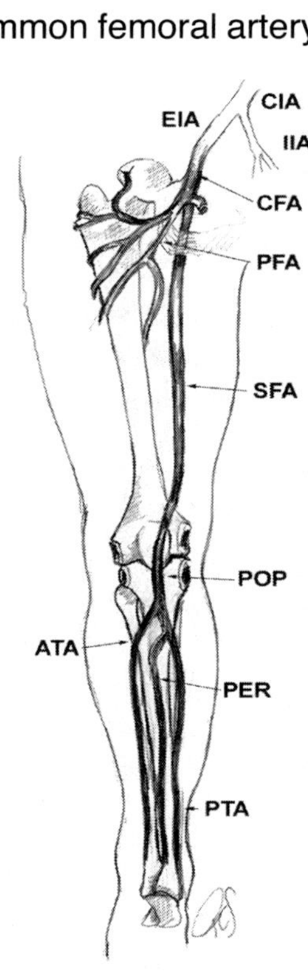

- Common femoral a. (CFA) - 2-3 cm distal to the groin, divides into profunda femoris artery and superficial femoral artery.
- Profunda femoris a. (deep femoral) (PFA) - supplies blood to the thigh muscles.
- Superficial femoral a. (SFA) - primarily a conduit of blood to the calf and lower leg. Courses through the adductor canal in the distal thigh to become the popliteal artery
- Popliteal a. (POP) - lies in the posterior aspect of the knee (popliteal fossa).
  - * Geniculate a.- a branch supplying the region of the knee.
  - * Gastrocnemius a.- first major branch of popliteal, supplies blood to the gastrocnemius muscles in the calf.

- Tibial Arteries
  - Anterior tibial a. (ATA) - first major tibial vessel branching from the distal popliteal; becomes the dorsalis pedis artery (DPA) at the crease of the ankle on the dorsum of the foot.
  - Tibio-peroneal trunk- a short segment that branches into the peroneal artery and the posterior tibial artery.
  - Posterior tibial a. (PTA) - courses along the tibia and lies posterior to the medial malleolus (MM) (medial ankle bone). Just distal to the MM, the PTA branches into the plantar arteries.
  - There are numerous communicating arteries between the PTA and the DPA in the ankle and foot.
- Microcirculation
  - Arterioles.
  - Capillaries.

Arterial Wall Anatomy

Intima

- The intima, or inner-most layer, consists of one layer of endothelial cells supported by an internal elastic lamina.
- Endothelium is a single layer of cells that lines the inner surface of the artery and is in contact with the intraluminal moving blood. It provides the following functions:

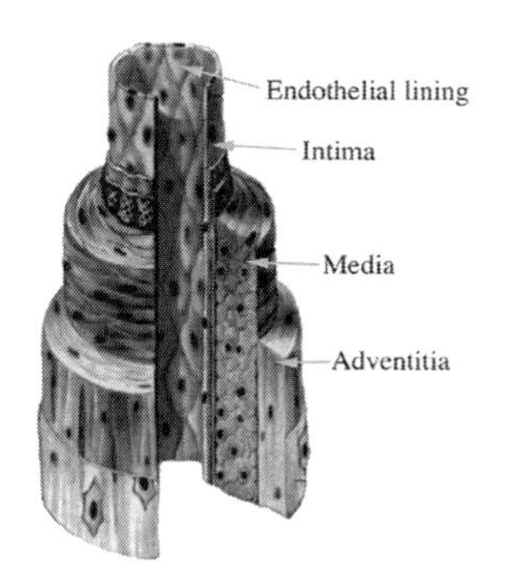

1. ***Permeability*** - it provides a barrier between blood and the artery wall that allows molecule

and nutrient exchange between blood plasma and the wall.

2. ***Antithrombogenic*** - it prevents platelets and monocytes (circulating white blood cells) from adhering to the artery wall.

3. ***Vasoreactivity*** - endothelial cells release endothelin, prostacyclin and Nitric Oxide that cause the artery wall (in the arterioles) to vasoconstrict and vasodilate.

Media

- The middle layer of the arterial wall consists primarily of smooth muscle cells, and allows rhythmic changes in the arterial size that occurs during the cardiac cycle.
- Collagen is also found in this area of the wall structure.
- The external elastic membrane lies between the media and the adventitia.

Adventitia

- The outer layer of the artery wall contains connective tissue and collagen, and the vasa vasorum, tiny blood vessels that supply the artery wall.

Arterioles

- These small arteries at the distal end of the arterial "tree" control blood flow into the capillary beds. They have the ability to constrict and reduce blood flow into tissue and muscle (primarily due to smooth muscle cell activity in the media), and to relax and allow more blood volume to pass.
- They play an important role in extremity blood flow, at rest and during exercise.

Capillaries

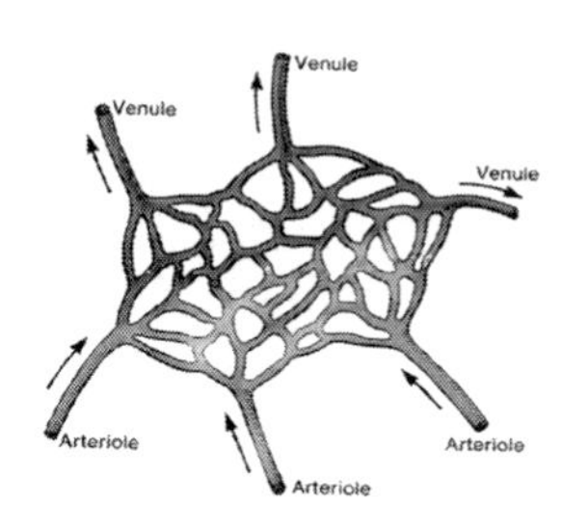

The smallest vessels in the circulatory system are the single-cell-walled capillaries. Small arterioles lead into the capillary beds, and venules carry blood back into the venous drainage system. The exchange of CO_2, O_2, and metabolic nutrients and metabolic waste takes place in the capillary beds. Flow through the capillary beds require a pressure gradient; high pressure on the arterial side and lower pressure in the venules.

A HEMODYNAMIC PRIMER

Hydrostatic Pressure (HP)

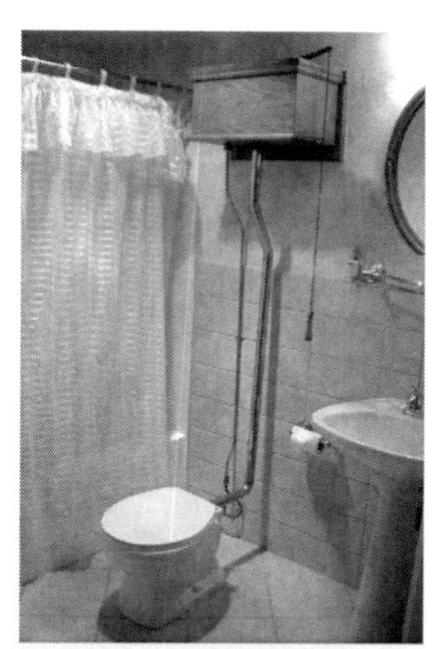

An effective use of hydostatic pressure!

The weight of the column of blood affects distal arterial and venous pressure when a person is sitting or standing. For each 12 inches (30.5 cm) of vertical distance below the heart, there is 22 mmHg of HP. For a person of 5' 10" in height (178 cm), the hydrostatic pressure at the ankle level is approximately 92 mmHg. This is in addition to the systolic blood pressure in the arterial system in the ankles. Ankle blood pressure determination should always be performed with the patient in a supine position to eliminate the effects of hydrostatic pressure.

Lower Extremity Normal Blood Flow at Rest

Cardiac output, intraluminal wall resistance, arterial wall compliance, and the dynamics of arteriolar vasoconstriction and vasodilation in the distal vascular beds control blood flow in the lower extremities.

In the basal or resting state, the arterioles are vasoconstricted as the demand for blood volume is low. Enabled by the closure of pre-capillary sphincters, arteriovenous shunting occurs in channels that bypass the capillary beds. Only 20-25% of capillaries are open in the skeletal muscles at rest. The arteriolar vasoconstriction contributes immensely to the high resistance found in the arterial system in the legs and arms.

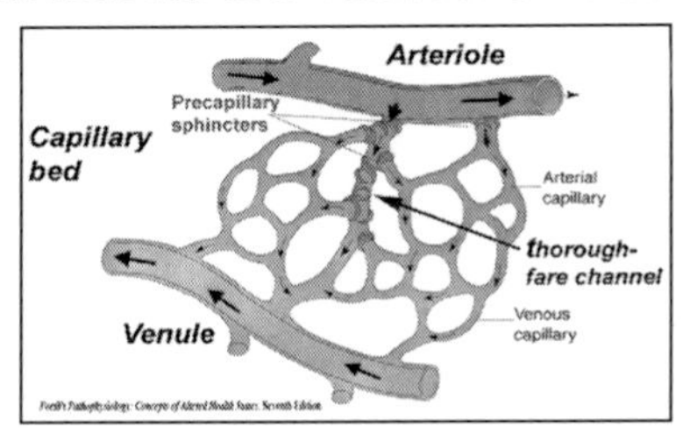

The effect of this resistance to blood flow is seen in Doppler waveforms. Blood flows forward towards the feet in systole, back towards the heart in early diastole, then forward again prior to the next systolic contraction. The display of this normal flow pattern is known as the triphasic or multiphasic waveform. On some normal patients the third component is absent; we just observe forward flow in systole, reverse flow in early diastole, and then no flow until the next cardiac cycle.

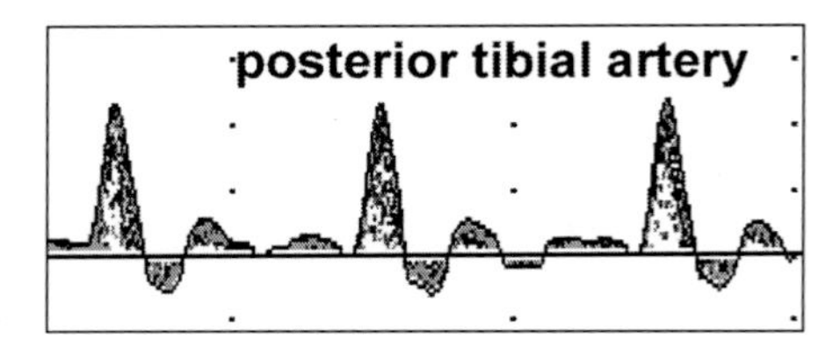

Lower extremity resting (low demand) perfusion summary:

⇒ Vasoconstriction in distal arterioles.

⇒ Arteriovenous shunting in muscle capillary beds.

⇒ Minimal blood flow to skeletal muscles.

⇒ Large blood volume exists in viscera and cerebral distributions.

⇒ High resistance in flow from the distal aorta to the arterioles.

Lower Extremity Blood Flow During Exercise

During exercise muscles need increased levels of oxygen and metabolites. The circulatory system also needs to remove more metabolic waste, carbon dioxide (CO_2) and lactic acid. Vasodilation (relaxation of smooth muscle cells in the artery wall) occurs in the arterioles as a product of local, nervous and hormonal regulatory mechanisms. There are a variety of "triggers" to cause vasodilation.

In normal individuals a substantial increase in blood flow volume occurs in the peripheral arteries during exercise. Arterial Doppler waveforms will change from a high-resistance pattern to a low-resistance pattern (see below).

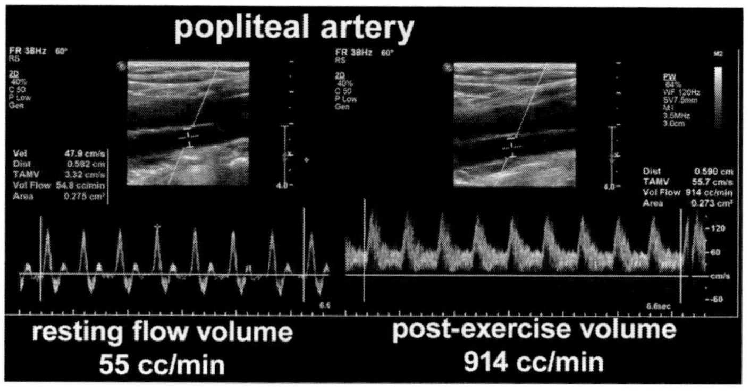

The left image above demonstrates a normal high-resistance popliteal artery waveform at rest. Flow volume was recorded at 55 ml/minute. After 3 minutes of exercise (walking on treadmill) the popliteal waveform has changed dramatically, and flow volume has increased to over 900 ml/min (cc/min).

Vasodilation in the lower vascular beds occurs quickly with the onset of exercise. The images below were obtained from a popliteal artery with a CW Doppler before and after just 5 toe raises (heel lifts).

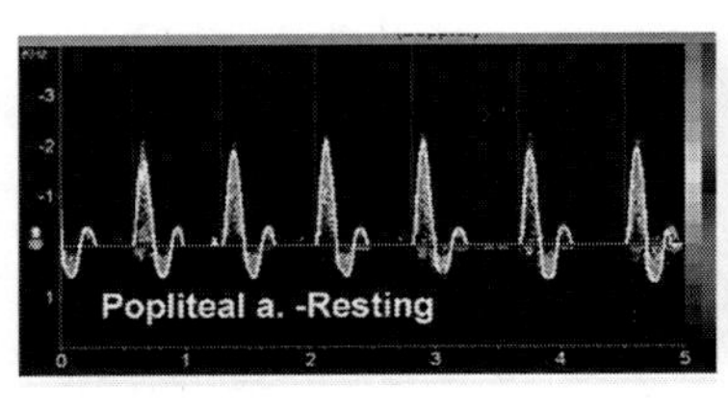

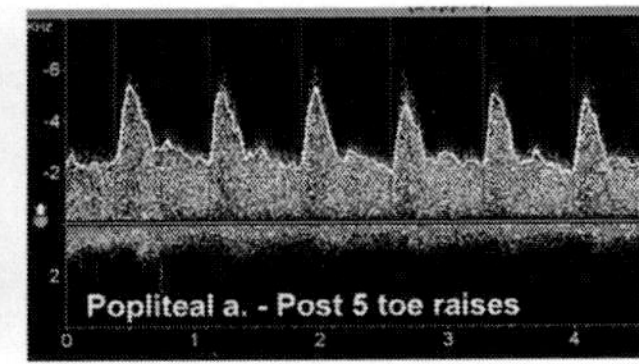

Despite the massive increase in blood flow volume when we exercise, blood pressure in the lower extremities, as measured at the ankle level, changes little. This phenomenon is explained by Poiseuille's law.

Poiseuille's law describes the relationship between flow, pressure gradient, viscosity, and length and radius of a tube. The simplified form can be expressed as:

$$Q = \frac{P}{R} \quad \text{Or} \quad Q \times R = P$$

Q= flow volume
R= resistance
P= distal pressure

During exercise, vasodilation occurs in the arterioles (radius increases) so peripheral resistance (R) decreases. As a result, flow volume (Q) increases. If the person exercising is normal (devoid of peripheral arterial disease), systolic pressure (P) in the legs and ankles remains about the same during exercise as it was before exercise. There may be a mild pressure increase linked to an increase in systemic pressure, but basically the ankle pressure does not change.

$$Q\uparrow \text{(increases)} \times R\downarrow \text{(decreases)} = \text{distal } P \text{ (no change)}$$

Lower Extremity Blood Flow: Patients with Arterial Occlusive Disease

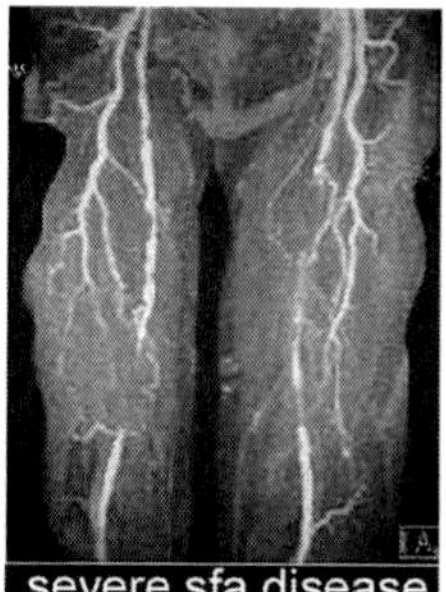
severe sfa disease

In patients with mild-moderate arterial occlusive disease, adequate distal perfusion may exist at rest when there is low demand. But during the high demand of exercise, the expected (and required) increase in blood volume to the skeletal muscles does not occur, or quantity is insufficient. Two scenarios contribute to inadequate volume, both are related to Poiseuille's law:

1. In the presence of occluded major arteries, the small-diameter collateral vessels cannot expand nor dilate, and the blood volume they can carry is limited. Note the stingy, small collaterals of the patient with bilateral SFA occlusions (above).

   As in a normal individual, vasodilation occurs in response to the need for more blood, and resistance decreases distally (a small change in the radius of a vessel has a major impact on resistance). When blood volume (Q) does not increase, distal pressure (P) falls. The skeletal muscles cannot obtain the necessary oxygen and metabolites to sustain exercise. When ankle pressure falls below 60 mmHg, transient muscle ischemia occurs and patients experience pain. See Poiseuille's formula below.

$$Q \text{ (no increase or decrease)} \times R \downarrow \text{(decreases)} = \text{distal } P \downarrow \text{(decreases)}$$

2. A second aspect of Poiseuille's law concerns the hemodynamic effect of flow volume change over a region of stenosis. In the words of Poiseuille:

> *"For a fixed narrowing with constant resistance, the pressure gradient through the narrowing is proportional to the flow through the narrowing. Small pressure gradients across a stenosis become larger with increased flow volume."*

So, for a patient with stenosis or multiple stenoses (versus total occlusion) increased flow volume during exercise causes a dramatic increase in the pressure gradient (pressure drop) over the stenosis. The diagram below illustrates a low flow and a high flow scenario over the same stenosis.

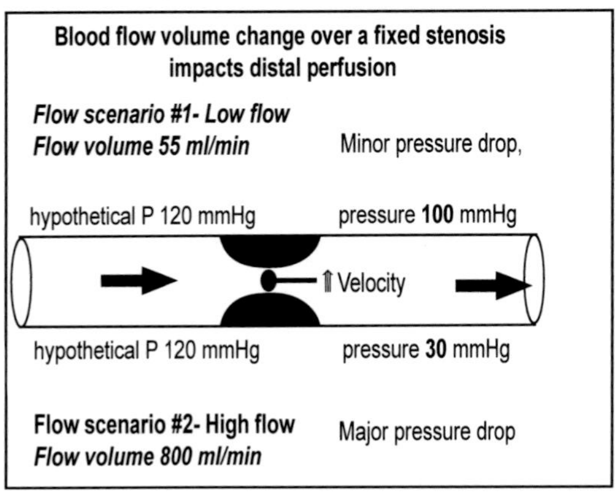

In both of the scenarios discussed, ankle pressure will decrease during exercise (there are exceptions of patients with well-developed collateral pathways). The figure on the right is a typical post-exercise ankle pressure graph demonstrating bilateral ankle pressure decrease after exercise, with slow recovery.

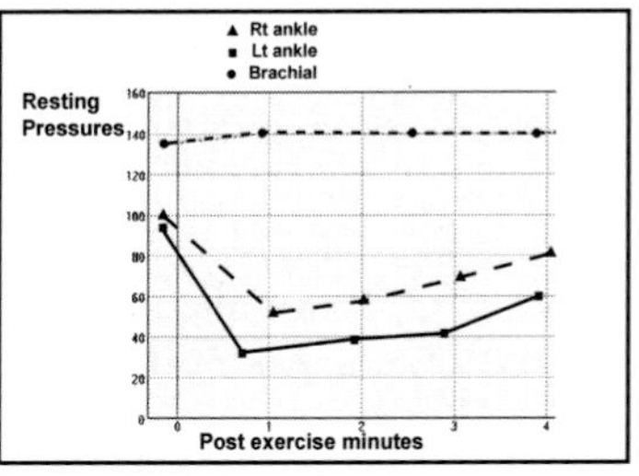

Patients may experience pain, fatigue, or cramping in the calf, thigh or buttock with exercise and this is known as <u>intermittent</u> claudication. Classically, the disability is progressive (the more they walk, the worse it gets) and is relieved by rest (cessation of exercise).

Vascular claudication usually takes place within the first few minutes of exercise and commonly limits the patient's walking distance to a city block or two, depending on the severity of disease and the extent of collateralization.

> *At our vascular lab in Colorado, referrals for lower arterial exams would increase in the fall season. Football fans would discover new-found claudication as they tried to ascend stairs to reach their seats in the upper decks at the local football stadiums!*

Patients with Severe PAD

In severe disease the arterioles will be chronically vasodilated at rest, and vasoreactivity absent. Often the Doppler waveforms will be persistently abnormal distal to the disease sites. Flow may be antegrade throughout the cardiac cycle and the waveform will lack the characteristic reversal in diastole.

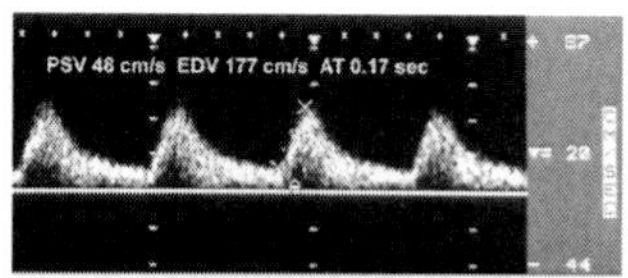

CFA distal to a severe aortic stenosis

On some patients we find a low-resistance waveform proximal to the disease level; again, this is due to vasodilation downstream.

The Doppler waveforms distal to severe occlusive disease may also be monophasic with a delayed rise time. In spectral Doppler this is called the tardus parvus waveform. As in this figure, flow occurs throughout diastole due to distal arteriole vasodilation. Often the pressure wave to too low to move blood in diastole, so we see small, diminished waveforms occurring just in systole.

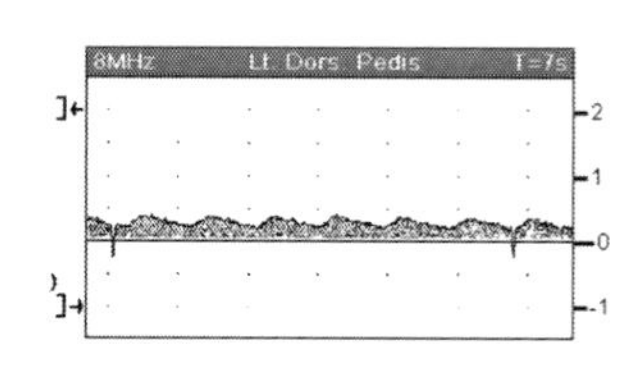

An understanding of normal and abnormal flow patterns helps us to identify PAD, judge severity, and locate the region of the occlusive disease.

Vasoreactivity also occurs in response to temperature, emotion (blushing), certain chemical reactions, and ischemia.

Hemodynamic Summary: Important Things to Remember

- Blood pressures in the ankles (also calves, and thighs) must be obtained with the patient supine (to eliminate the effects of hydrostatic pressure).
- Doppler waveforms (and pulse volume recordings) in the legs and arms are 'shaped" primarily by resistance in the distal arterioles.
- Most patients with PAD are asymptomatic at rest; they become symptomatic when they exercise.
- Some patients will have vascular disease that will not be detected with physiologic testing performed at rest. If claudication symptoms exist, this subset of patients should be exercised and retested.

References

1. Wikipedia. http://en.wikipedia.org/wiki/Atherosclerosis

CHAPTER 2: INSTRUMENTATION-TOOLS OF THE TRADE

This chapter will review instrumentation and methods specific to indirect physiologic testing.

DOPPLER ULTRASOUND

One of the main tools of physiologic testing is continuous-wave Doppler, or CW Doppler. In its simplest form, it's used as a Doppler "stethoscope" to detect the present or absence of blood flow, and to note sound characteristics associated with flow patterns. More advanced applications include recording Doppler waveforms to assess blood flow patterns associated with different disease levels, and to observe flow direction. Pulsed-wave Doppler (PW Doppler), a more sophisticated system, is used on duplex ultrasound systems and is not used in indirect physiologic testing.

THE DOPPLER SHIFT - BASIC PRINCIPLES

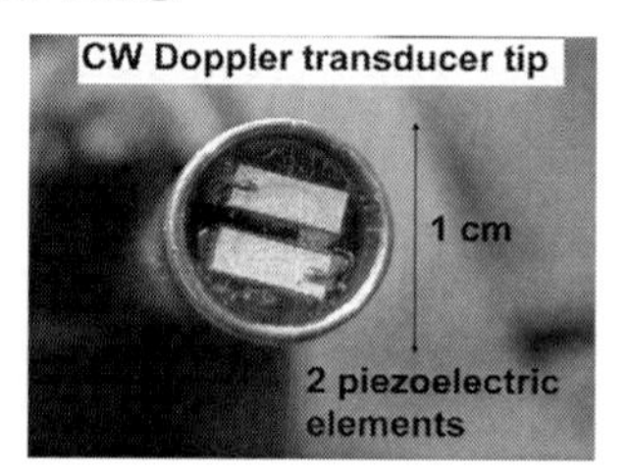

In diagnostic ultrasound the echo Doppler principle is used to detect blood flow. A transducer with 2 piezoelectric elements is used to transmit a high frequency ultrasound signal into tissue, and to receive the returning echo.

Frequency

- Sound consists of pressure waves.
- Frequency is the number of wave cycles per second. Frequency is expressed in hertz, 1 sound wave or cycle per second = 1 hertz or Hz.
- The range of frequency that humans can hear is 20 Hz-20,000 Hz, or 20 kHz.

- For diagnostic ultrasound, Doppler frequency is between 2.0 - 10 MHz (megahertz). This is beyond the range of human hearing.
- Sound is absorbed or attenuated as it travels through air, water and tissue. Low frequency sound has better penetration and travels farther than high frequency sound. For example, your car shakes from the big bass sounds coming from the kid's car behind you at the stoplight! You don't hear the high frequency notes, as they don't carry far, just the lower frequencies of bass notes.
- Doppler depth penetration is related to transmitted frequency; the lower the frequency, the better the penetration. Doppler sensitivity is also related to transmitted frequency; the higher the frequency, the better the sensitivity (ability to detect low flow), but, at the expense of penetration.
- Most physiologic testing systems provide a high frequency Doppler transducer (8 or 10 MHz) and a low frequency transducer (4 or 5 MHz). The former is used for assessing arteries at the ankle level, and the latter for deeper vessels like the femoral and popliteal arteries. As will be discussed later, a single high-frequency CW Doppler is sufficient for ABIs and segmental pressure acquisition. If segmental Doppler waveforms of the lower extremities are to be included in your protocol, then both transducers should be used.
- The frequency of the transducer is dictated by the size (thickness) of the piezoelectric elements.

Piezoelectric Elements

- Piezoelectric elements are made from ceramic material with a special property to enable them to transmit sound. A single element within the transducer is stimulated with electricity (voltage); this causes the ceramic material to oscillate and transmit a high-frequency sound signal.

- The sound waves travel into the tissue and reflect back to the piezoelectric element in the transducer. The returning echo vibrates the piezo element and creates a voltage.
- The returning echo is analyzed to see if the frequency (number of waves or cycles per second) has changed, i.e., the Doppler system compares the frequency of the transmitted signal to the frequency of the returning echo. The difference between the two is called the **Doppler Shift.**

The Doppler Shift

When the Doppler "beam" crosses moving red blood cells within an artery or a vein, the returning frequency (the echo) will change. The transmitted frequency of the CW Doppler transducer is too high for us to hear, and the returning frequency is also too high to hear, but the Doppler shift frequency falls within our hearing range.

The diagram below illustrates the Doppler shift related to blood flow towards and away from the transducer.

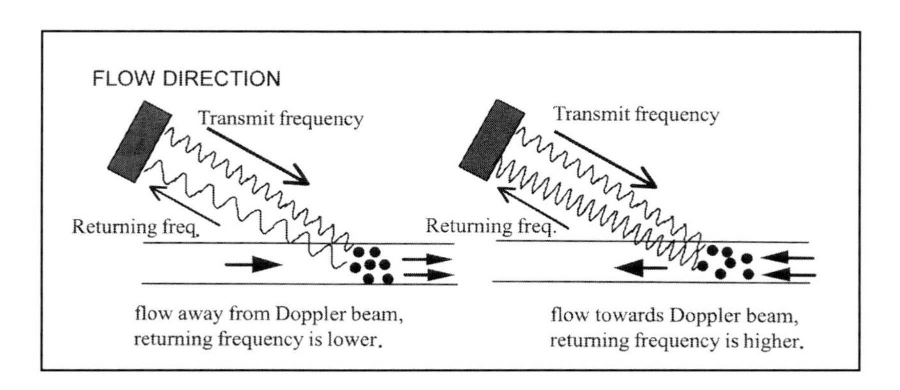

In the both examples the transmitted frequency is the same.

⇒ If blood cells are moving away from the direction of the

transmitted Doppler signal, the returning echo will be lower in frequency (fewer cycles per second).

⇒ If blood flow is towards the Doppler beam, the echo will be higher in frequency.

⇒ Generally, flow moving towards the Doppler beam is displayed above the baseline in the Doppler recording (this is called a "positive" shift). Blood flow moving away from the Doppler beam is a "negative" shift and is displayed below baseline.

⇒ If the returning frequency is the same as the transmit frequency, which would occur if there is no motion or movement, there is no Doppler shift.

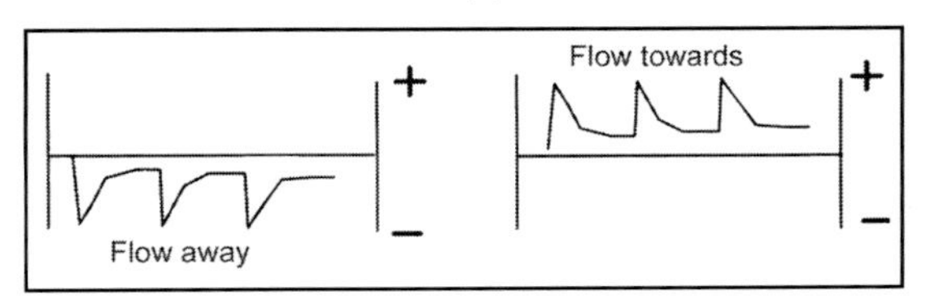

Two major things affect the frequency shift (what we hear and see on the Doppler display).

1. The speed of the blood cells; the faster the blood speed, the higher the Doppler shift. Arterial flow usually has a higher frequency sound than venous flow as the former is traveling at a much greater speed.

2. The Doppler "angle to flow", i.e., the angle created by the Doppler beam as it intersects the vessel. The angle business is very important.

Theoretically, the maximum Doppler shift occurs at a zero degree angle to flow (rarely achieved). The worst Doppler shift occurs at 90 degrees to flow (easily obtained!), see below.

CW-DOPPLER METHODS

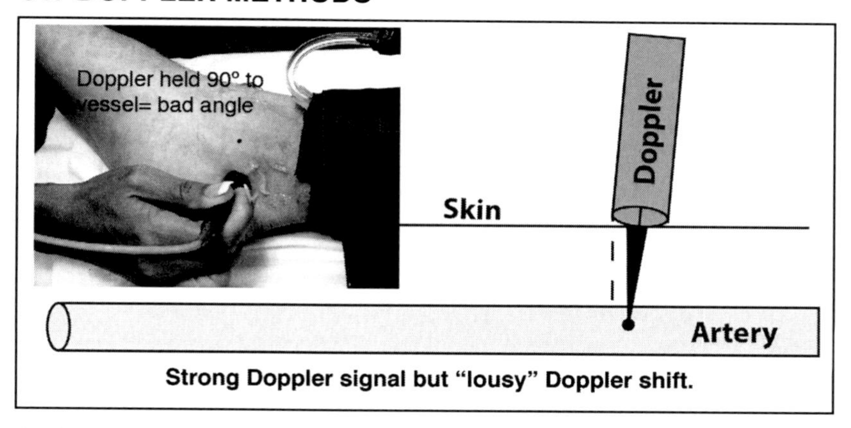

Strong Doppler signal but "lousy" Doppler shift.

In the image above, the Doppler transducer is held perpendicular to the skin over the posterior tibial artery and just posterior to the medial malleolus (the large medial bone of the ankle). This will result is a poor Doppler shift of low frequency due to the high angle. The resulting Doppler waveform will be of low amplitude and probably non-diagnostic.

If the transducer is "laid back" too far to create a small angle to the skin, the Doppler signal may be too weak to be diagnostic; in fact, you might not hear any Doppler signal even though you're over the artery, see diagram below.

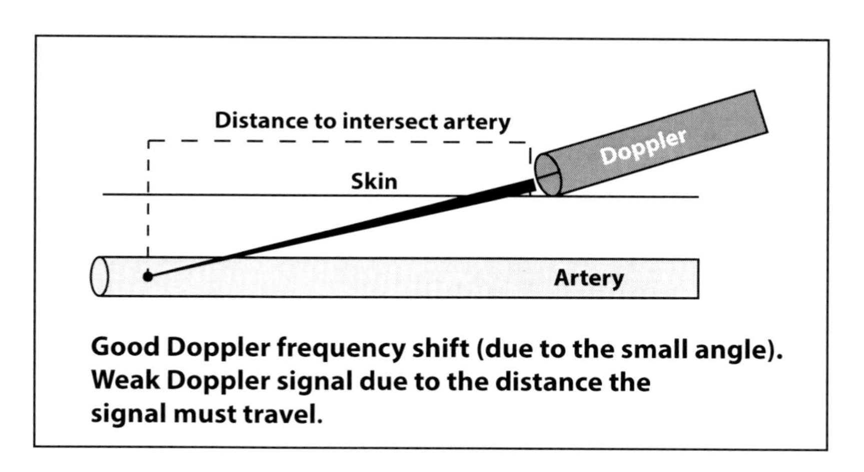

Good Doppler frequency shift (due to the small angle). Weak Doppler signal due to the distance the signal must travel.

In the diagram above the ultrasound beam must travel a long distance, down and back, to intersect the arterial flow. This results in a weak Doppler signal.

The CW Doppler transducer should be held at a **45 - 60° angle** to the skin and pointed along the long axis of the artery. This will provide a good compromise between signal strength and Doppler shift, see below.

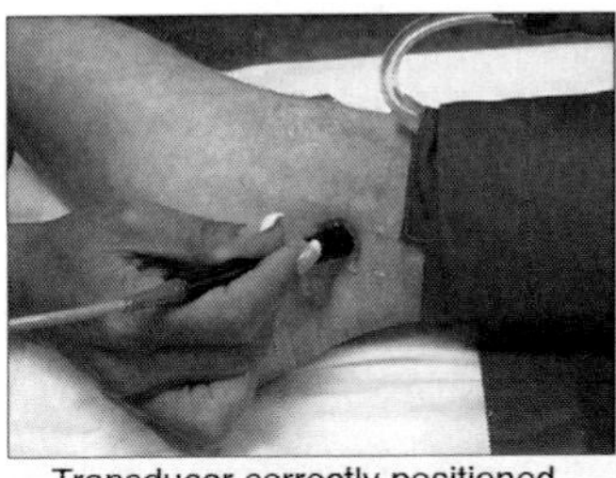

Transducer correctly positioned at a 45-60° angle to skin.

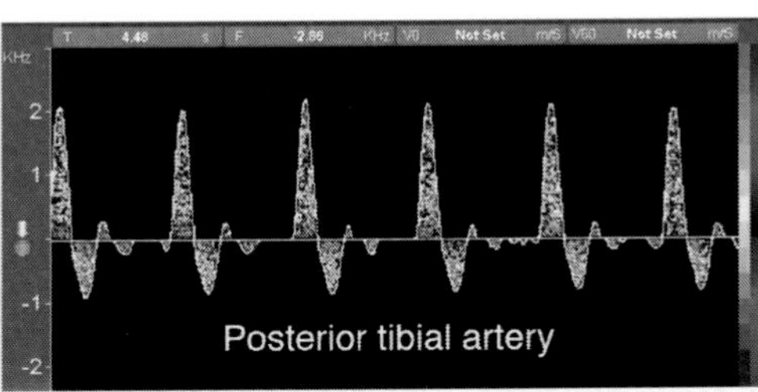

This is a normal, multiphasic waveform obtained with a CW Doppler (with FFT spectral display), the transducer is held at a 45° angle.

Compare the normal spectral waveform above, to the one below. The one below is obtained from a nearly 90° angle.

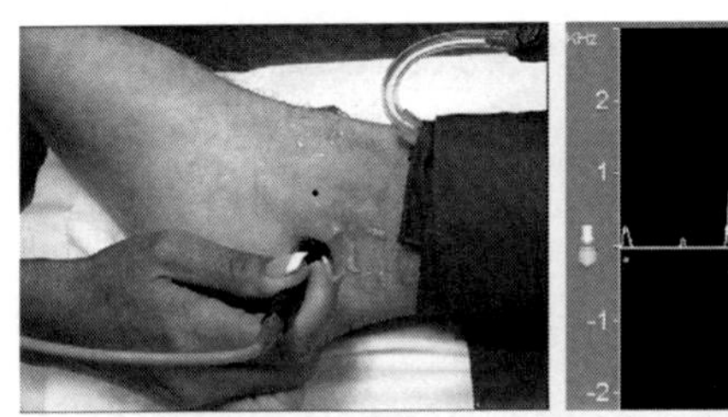

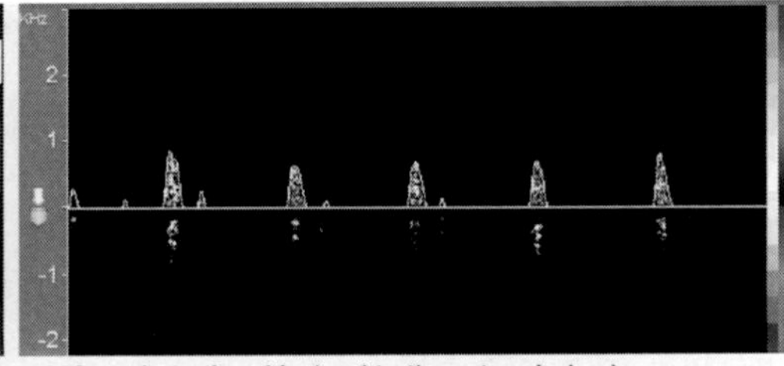

The Doppler probe is held at nearly a 90° angle to the skin (and to the artery below). The resulting waveform, from the same normal PTA , is poor, contains "noise" and would be judged to be abnormal.

The most common mistake in obtaining a Doppler waveform, whether for pressure assessment or waveform analysis, is holding the Doppler at an inappropriate angle (too steep).

Because the transducer is held at an angle to the skin, you must use a good amount of acoustic gel at the tip of the transducer to maintain contact. There is a tendency for sonographers to minimize the amount of gel (Yo, it's pretty inexpensive!!). In general and vascular ultrasound, linear array transducers are held FLAT against the skin, so only a small amount of gel is needed for good coupling. This is not the case with CW Doppler.

Centering the Doppler Beam

The Doppler beam must also be centered over the artery. Once you acquire a Doppler signal (at the appropriate angle to the skin) ***slowly*** move the probe across the skin until you find the strongest signal. You won't know if you have "the strongest signal" unless you sweep the transducer all the way across the vessel. Slide the probe across until you lose the sound, then sweep back to the location of the strongest signal.

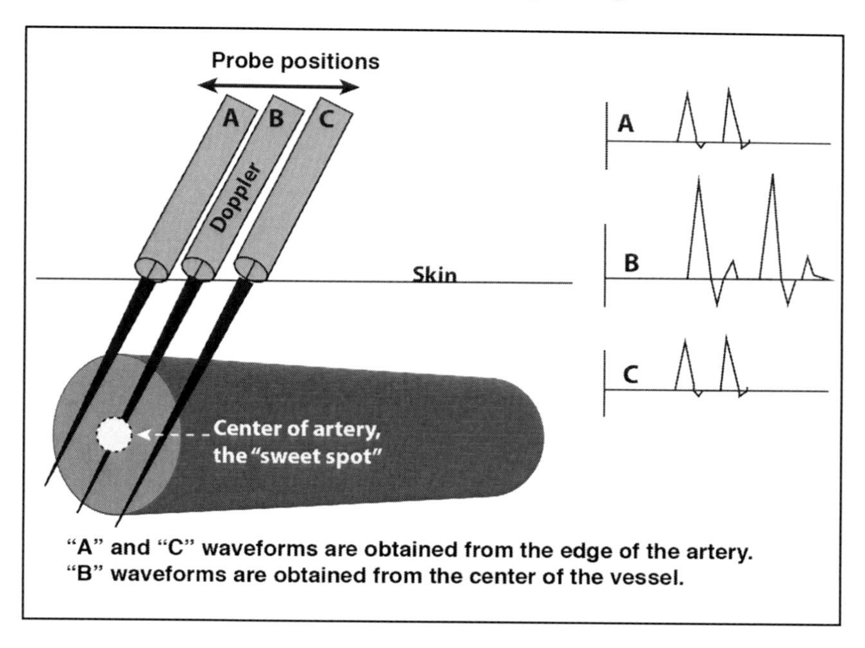

"A" and "C" waveforms are obtained from the edge of the artery.
"B" waveforms are obtained from the center of the vessel.

When acquiring pressures, you're less likely to slide off the artery if you start with the beam centered.

THE DOPPLER DISPLAY

Some small hand-held CW Doppler devices only provide an audible signal, with perhaps an indicator for flow direction. For physiologic testing, waveforms are displayed from the Doppler frequency information. There are 2 methods for generating waveforms in physiologic testing.

1. Analog Processing, or Analog Doppler

Also called zero-crossing detection, this method displays a single-line trace representing average velocity (it's actually an average frequency trace). This is the most popular method found in physiologic testing equipment and it provides adequate information; it's also less expensive to produce than the FFT spectral Doppler method.

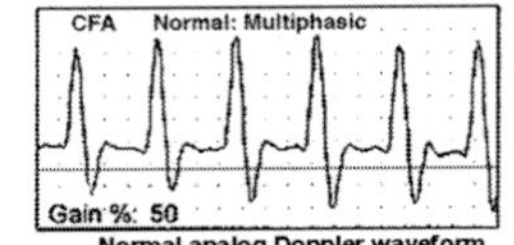

Normal analog Doppler waveform,

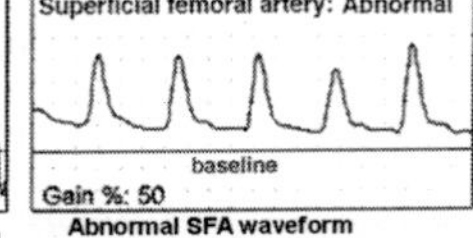

Abnormal SFA waveform

- The sweep rate affects the appearance of the waveforms; for Doppler waveform acquisition and storage a 2.5 or 5 second time sweep is customary. For pressure acquisition, where the actual waveform is not saved or stored, the sweep time is usually much longer.
- A limitation of analog Doppler occurs when there is more than one vessel in the beam path of the Doppler. Unlike pulsed-wave Doppler, which is specific for a predefined depth, CW Doppler will detect any movement or blood flow that occurs within the beam path, up to the limits of the depth penetration.

⇒ Because major deep veins lie adjacent to major arteries, it's not uncommon to detect a vein and an artery in the same Doppler signal. Because the two different signals are averaged into one analog display, waveform distortion can occur.

> If a venous signal is corrupting the arterial Doppler waveform, try to change transducer positions to eliminate the venous signal. Also, the venous flow can be stopped by having the patient hold their breath for a few moments.

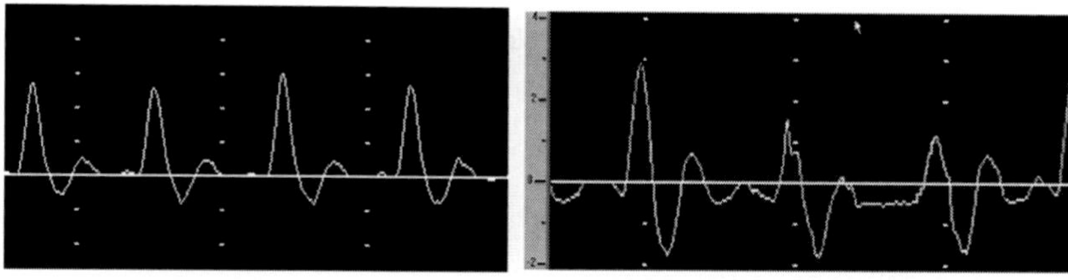

PTA normal waveform **PTA waveform with venous interference.**

In the graphic above, a normal posterior tibial artery analog waveform is shown on the left. The waveform on the right is corrupted by the effect of the posterior tibial vein that falls in the beam path.

2. Spectral Doppler Display

Also known as Fast Fourier Transform (FFT), this display is available on some CW Doppler systems, but it's not as common as analog Doppler. This processing method is similar to that found on color duplex ultrasound systems. Although more expensive to produce, it has the advantage of displaying peak frequencies, and it can display arterial and venous flow simultaneously. Some systems have a colorized spectral display, others are in gray-scale.

CW Doppler Spectral Waveforms

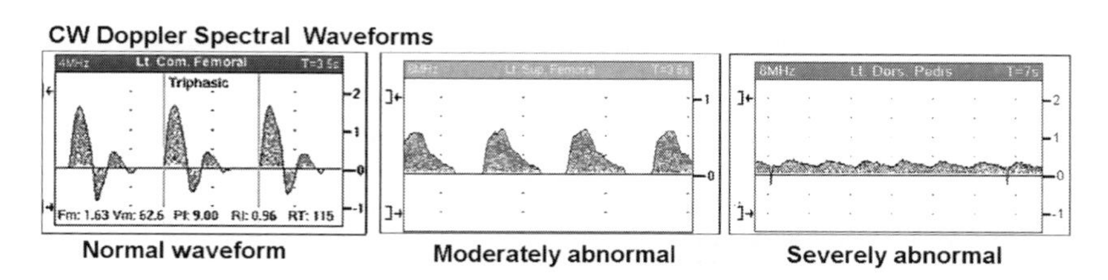

Normal waveform **Moderately abnormal** **Severely abnormal**

- In duplex ultrasound, flow velocity can be calculated because the actual Doppler angle to flow can be measured.

Accurate velocity measurements cannot be accomplished with hand-held CW Doppler methods, (both analog and spectral Doppler) as the true Doppler angle is unknown.

- Because the Doppler angle to flow is not known, and because frequency shifts vary with Doppler angle, CW Doppler waveform measurements are not quantitative. Waveforms are evaluated qualitatively for normal and abnormal patterns of flow.

Doppler Scale

The appearance of the Doppler waveform is affected by the *gain* control in analog Doppler and by the gain and scale controls in spectral Doppler.

- A normal waveform can be made to appear abnormal if the scale is adjusted incorrectly.
- Some laboratories prefer to use the same gain settings at all locations when acquiring Doppler segmental waveforms. This can result in the PTA and DPA waveforms appearing much smaller than waveforms from the CFA, SFA, and popliteal sites.
- This author prefers to use a gain or scale that optimizes the size of the waveform; the amplitude is less important than being able to evaluate the shape of the waveform. However, it's recommended to use the same scale or gain at the contralateral site.

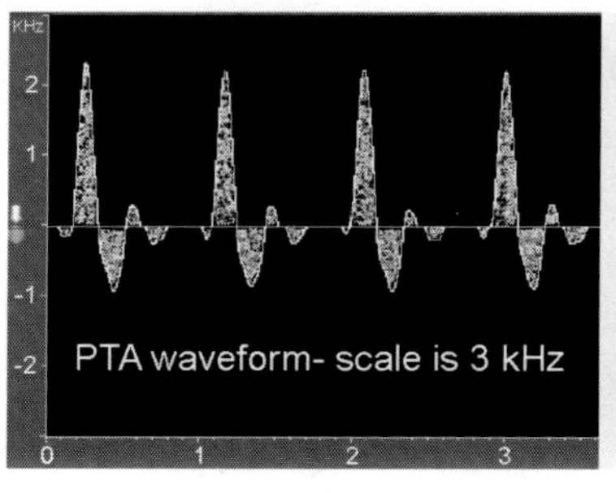

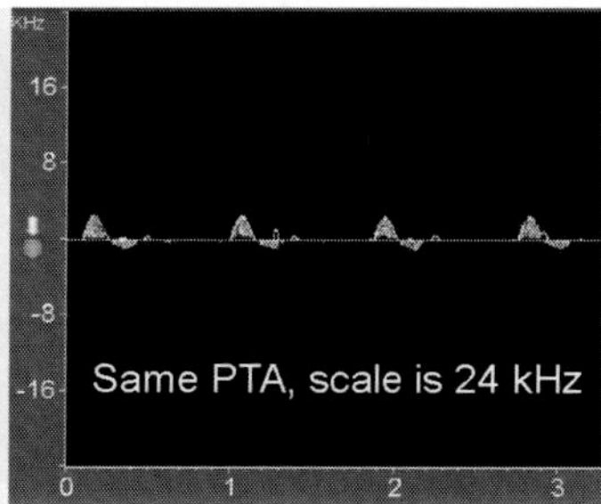

The Doppler waveforms above are from the same artery. The waveform on the left was obtained with the correct scale. The waveform on the right was obtained with a scale that is set too high; consequently, the waveform is too small to be of diagnostic value.

- Although CW Doppler waveforms may go “off-scale”, it's due to inappropriate scale settings rather than aliasing. The aliasing artifact that is commonly experienced in PW Doppler, advantageously does not occur in CW Doppler.

Doppler Summary

- CW Doppler is used as an ultrasonic “stethoscope” when acquiring blood pressures. When combined with a pressure cuff and a sphygmomanometer, the audible signal and the waveforms are used to measure systolic blood pressure.
- You cannot obtain diastolic pressure with a Doppler device.
- CW Doppler can be used to obtain and record arterial waveforms from various sites on the arms and legs. Pattern recognition skills can be used to determine normal versus abnormal flow patterns.
- Use an 8 - 10 MHZ CW Doppler for the radial, brachial posterior tibial, and dorsalis pedis arteries.
- For deeper vessels, use a 4-5 MHZ transducer.
- Hold the transducer 45-60° angle to the skin, align the probe along the long axis of the vessel.
- Point or aim the transducer towards the direction of flow, (blood flow should be coming towards the Doppler beam).
- You need a steady hand, so hold the transducer in a fashion that will allow your fingers and hand to rest on the foot, leg or arm so that the probe will not slide off the artery below.

- Use a sufficient amount of acoustic coupling gel (the thick stuff that doesn't "run" is preferred).
- Always sweep the Doppler beam across the artery (slowly) to maximize signal strength (at the center of the artery). This applies for both pressure testing and waveform acquisition.
- Use appropriate scale/gain to optimize the waveform appearance; make them big!

PULSE VOLUME RECORDING (PVR) (VPR)

This is a form of air or pneumo-plethysmography (pleth is mog grau phie). The method generates waveforms that can be assessed for the presence or absence of arterial occlusive disease.

Segmental air plethysmography, or pulse volume recording, is used to measure the change in limb volume related to each cardiac cycle. Pulse Volume Recording is abbreviated as PVR. Parks Medical Electronics uses the term Volume Pulse Recording, or VPR.

PVR: How It Works

- Blood volume in the legs and arms increases in systole and decreases in diastole. Consequently, the girth of the limb increases and decreases with the cardiac cycle.
- Pressure cuffs are placed around the limbs, usually bilaterally. The cuffs are inflated to a fixed pressure (65 mmHg ± 5 mmHg).

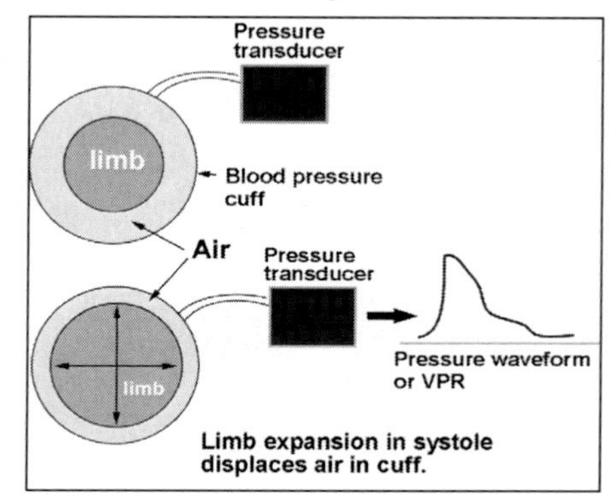

Limb expansion in systole displaces air in cuff.

- The air pressure is held steady and not "bled down" as in pressure acquisition. As the limb expands in systole as a result of increased blood volume, the air pressure within the cuff increases; in diastole it decreases. This pulsating change in cuff pressure is recorded on the plethysmograph, a sensitive pressure transducer that's connected to a digital recording system. Modern systems can store PVR data for printout at the completion of the exam. Historically, PVRs were recorded on a paper strip-chart recorder.

- Some manufacturers list the volume of air injected into each cuff for contralateral comparison. Amplitude differences can occur in the waveforms if there is a significant volume discrepancy. For this reason it's important that the cuffs be wrapped as snugly as possible, and uniformly from side to side.
- PVR waveforms provide a profile of global limb perfusion, including the effect of collateralization (unlike Doppler waveforms that provide a profile of specific artery flow).
- PVR cuffs are the same as those used for acquiring blood pressures.
- PVRs are usually performed bilaterally.
- In the lower extremities, PVRs can be obtained from the thigh, calf, ankle, metatarsal, and great toe locations.
- PVRs can also be used to assess upper extremity perfusion, including digits.
- Waveform assessment is subjective and not quantitative.

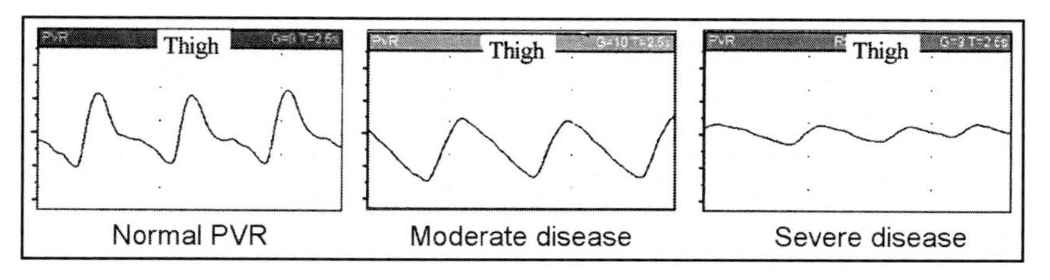

The PVRs above demonstrate the following:

A normal PVR waveform has a sharp upslope and a prominent reflected wave (also called the dicrotic notch) in late systole and early diastole in the downslope.

A moderately abnormal PVR has a rounded peak, no reflected wave and a pronounced decrease in amplitude.

A severely abnormal PVR is of low amplitude, reflective wave is absent, and waveform might even be "flatline".

PVR limitations: in the presence of severe proximal (inflow) disease, PVR accuracy in predicting distal disease is reduced. Also, PVRs require good patient cooperation; limb motion or tremor adversely affects waveform contour. Patients should be instructed not to move or talk during this test.

Pulse volume recording is easy to perform and the only skill required is the ability to wrap the pressure cuffs snugly (See QR code demo Chapter 3, page 38).

PHOTO-PLETHYSMOGRAPHY (PPG)

PPG is an important tool for evaluating digit perfusion. The device is small, and it can be attached to the fingers or toes with a clip that fits around the digit, a Velcro® strap, or double-stick transparent tape.

- The PPG sensor transmits infrared light into the skin, some of the light is absorbed by red blood cells and some is reflected back to the sensor.
- A waveform is generated that allows an assessment of cutaneous blood flow based on the shape of the waveform.

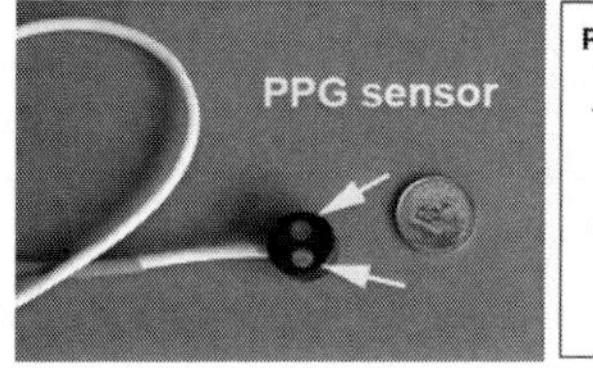

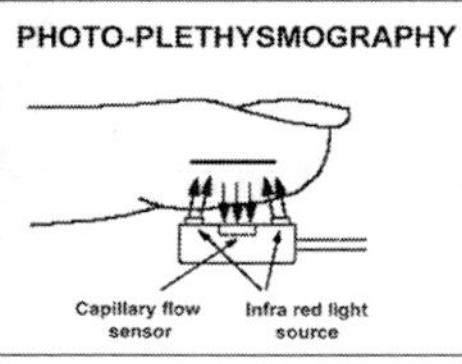

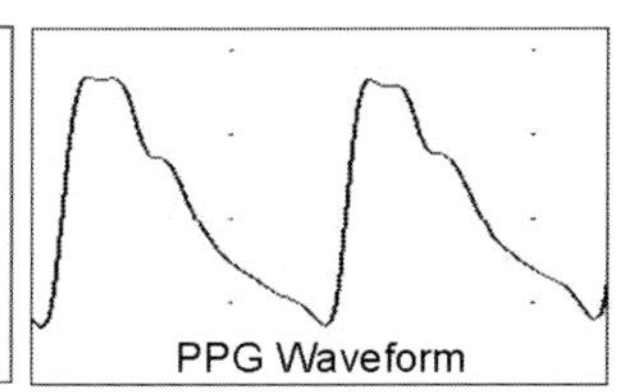

- PPG can also be used for pressure measurements. The waveform (processing modified with a slow sweep speed) is used as the "marker" for the return of systolic pressure. It replaces the Doppler for that purpose and is very good for obtaining digit pressures.

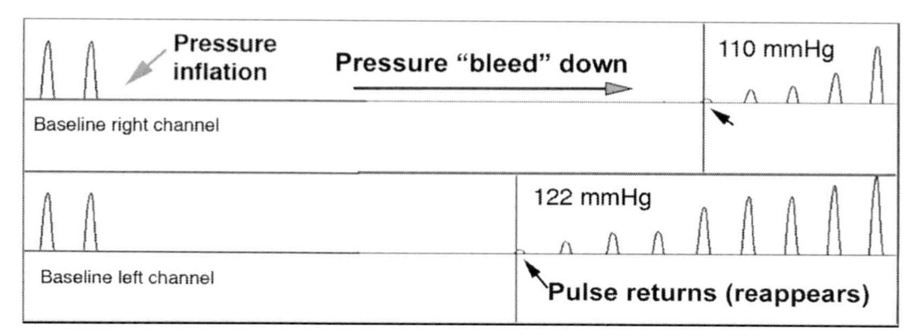

PPG bilateral pressure sequence

The graphic above demonstrates bilateral digit pressure acquisition using PPG. Baseline waveforms are established, then digit pressure cuffs are inflated to supra-systolic pressure to obliterate the waveforms. Pressure is "bled down" until the pulses reappear on both digits. Cuffs are deflated and the first returning pulse of each digit identified. A vertical line, linked to the pressure manometer, is moved to the first pulse on each digit and systolic pressures are recorded. Alternatively, depending on the system, the waveforms are scrolled to a side line that represents the pressure reading.

This method can also be used to obtain ankle and other limb pressures. However, in 2001 CMS (Medicare) revised guidelines for noninvasive physiologic testing to exclude this method for obtaining ankle blood pressures. The new guidelines require that Doppler pressure measurements be obtained from both the PTA and the DPA, and this cannot be accomplished with the PPG pressure method. This also excludes oscillometric pressure methods for ABIs.

Clinical applications of PPG include:

⇒ Digit evaluation for small vessel occlusive disease in the fingers and toes.

⇒ Thoracic outlet testing.

⇒ Cold immersion testing for Raynaud's Syndrome.

⇒ Great toe pressures.

⇒ Finger pressures.

⇒ Penile pressures.

⇒ Venous insufficiency testing.

TREADMILL

Treadmill stress testing is used for a subset of patients suspected of having peripheral arterial disease (PAD). Those patients that either have mild - moderate disease or those with borderline resting physiologic studies.

The treadmill should have these features:

⇒ Adjustable speed from 1-2.5 MPH.

⇒ Sturdy hand rail.

⇒ Adjustable elevation, up to 10 percent grade.

⇒ It should be located in the same room that physiologic arterial testing is performed.

⇒ Must have a conveniently located stop switch.

Other useful items for vascular testing:

- Clear plastic wrap, or Tegaderm for covering ulcers and wounds prior to applying blood pressure cuffs.
- Acoustic gel for Doppler transducer.
- Electric heating pad for upper digit testing.
- A basin for cold water for cold immersion testing (upper extremity digits).
- Disinfectant for cleaning cuffs.

CHAPTER 3: ARTERIAL PHYSIOLOGIC TESTING: LOWER EXTREMITIES

Indirect physiologic testing of the lower extremities is performed to detect hemodynamically significant arterial occlusive disease, i.e., disease severe enough to reduce arterial pressure and perfusion distally, whether at rest or during exercise. Stenoses which may cause focal velocity increase but which do not impact downstream perfusion are not readily detected with these methods.

THE GOALS OF LOWER EXTREMITY PHYSIOLOGIC TESTING

1. To determine if there is objective evidence for arterial occlusive disease.
   - ⇒ Palpation of limb pulses and patient history are subjective and often unreliable.
2. If disease is present, to determine the severity.
3. If disease is present, is it causing the patient's symptoms?
   - ⇒ In patients with combined neuropathy and peripheral arterial disease, physiologic testing (with stress testing) may be the only objective way to determine which condition is causing the patient's symptoms.[1]
4. If disease is present, to determine the region of disease (aortoiliac, femoro-popliteal, popliteal-tibial, or multi-segment disease).

In addition, ankle and toe pressures are useful in predicting whether sufficient perfusion exists to heal ulceration and foot wounds.[2]

The Advantages of Physiologic Testing:

⇒ It's simple to perform and requires only a short learning curve.

⇒ The testing time is short, ranging from 20 - 45 minutes for a complete bilateral exam.

⇒ It's accurate for detecting hemodynamically significant disease.

⇒ It provides objective, quantitative physiologic information.

⇒ The instrumentation is relatively inexpensive compared to ultrasound systems.

Normal test results at rest and following exercise or post-reactive hyperemia rule out hemodynamically significant arterial occlusive disease (> 60% diameter stenosis). These methods have high sensitivity and specificity for the presence of symptomatic atherosclerotic disease.

Limitations include the inability to identify the precise location of stenosis or occlusion. Diagnoses tend to be generalized in regard to the region (aortoiliac, femoro-popliteal, popliteal-tibial) and to disease severity (mild, moderate, severe). Physiologic testing will not detect minor levels of diffuse atherosclerotic disease.

Indirect Physiologic Test Methods

- Pulse Volume Recordings (PVR) or Volume Pulse Recording (VPR).
- Doppler analog waveform analysis, or Doppler spectral analysis.
- Segmental Limb Pressures (SLP) and calculated Ankle/Brachial Indices (ABI) and Toe/Brachial Indices (TBI).

- Exercise stress test (treadmill or toe raises).

Diagnostic laboratories may perform all of the above tests, or may use a specific combination, e.g., SLP, PVR, and exercise stress test, or they may substitute Doppler waveforms for PVRs.

PATIENT HISTORY

Prior to any arterial testing, it's important to obtain a good patient history, including a complete description of the current symptoms.

> Prior to testing, you need to be sure you're performing the correct exam. There is some confusion with referring parties as to the symptoms of arterial versus venous disease. You may receive an order for an arterial exam but the symptoms are those of deep venous thrombosis (DVT), or vice versa. A full segmental arterial exam on someone with undiagnosed acute DVT could cause a fatal pulmonary embolus. *Do not perform an arterial exam on a patient suspected of having acute deep venous thrombosis.*

Pertinent questions should include:

- Do you have leg pain when you walk, and if so, is it in both legs?
- What part of your leg hurts (calf, thigh, buttock, or hip)?
- Which leg is the worse?
- Is the pain progressive and does it stop you from walking?
- How many blocks can you walk before you cannot go on?
- Does the pain go away when you stop walking?
- How long have you been having this problem?
- Do you have pain in your feet or toes at night?

- Have you ever had a bypass graft, a stent, or arterial operation, and if so, what type?

Risk Factors Should Be Noted

- Is the patient a smoker, and if so, how many packs are smoked per day and for how many years?
- Does the patient have diabetes mellitus (DM) and does he/she take insulin?
- Has the patient ever had a stroke (CVA), transient ischemic attack (TIA), or myocardial infarction (MI) (heart attack)?
- Is there a family history of CVA, or MI?
- Does the patient have hypertension (HT)?
- Does the patient have hyperlipidemia (high cholesterol levels)?

Palpation of Pulses - Optional

Although palpation of peripheral pulses has traditionally been part of the physical examination, it is subjective information. Limb pressure measurements are more objective and reliable that pulse palpation.

If limb pulses are palpated, they are rated in the following manner. Some institutions use a 5 gradation scale, but 4 levels will be described here:
0 = no pulse.
1^+ = weak pulse.
2^+ = normal pulse.
3^+ = very strong pulse or aneurysmal pulses (this is when you can observe your hand moving up and down with each pulsation).

Pulses may be palpated at the following sites:
- Common femoral artery (CFA) in the groin.
- Popliteal artery in the popliteal fossa behind the knee.

- Dorsalis pedis artery (DPA) on top of the foot.
- Posterior tibial artery (PTA) below the medial malleolus on the medial side of the ankle.

NOTE: Pedal pulses may not be palpated if ankle pressures are below 100 mmHg. Popliteal pulses in many normals are not palpated due to the depth of the artery. CFA pulses are important in the diagnosis of inflow (aorto-iliac) disease versus infrainguinal (below the groin) disease.

PHYSICAL SIGNS OF DISEASE

Look for physical signs of disease:

⇒ Pallor.

⇒ Extremity coldness.

⇒ Dependent rubor (redness when leg is below heart level, limb blanching when elevated above heart level).

⇒ Cyanotic toes.

⇒ Ulceration on lower leg/foot/toes.

⇒ Non-healing wounds on feet and toes.

⇒ Blue toe syndrome: a symptom of embolization.

⇒ Gangrene.

In recent years the level of awareness of what symptoms indicate a venous examination versus an arterial exam has decreased. The federal agency governing Medicare, CMS, has stated, “the provider of the service is ultimately responsible for the appropriateness of the examination”. The technologist/ sonographer must be aware of what constitutes appropriate indications for venous and arterial symptoms. If the indications do not match the ordered examination, the order should be confirmed with the ordering physician. In many states, reimbursement for an arterial and venous exam performed on the same patient for the same indication is not allowed.

The table below is a limited comparison of symptoms; deep venous thrombosis (DVT) versus peripheral arterial disease (PAD).

COMPARISON OF SYMPTOMS: ACUTE DVT VS. ARTERIAL	
Symptoms of Acute DVT	**Symptoms of PAD**
Acute, persistent pain: thigh or calf	Chronic symptoms, developed over years
Persistent limb swelling	No swelling
Local tenderness in calf	Intermittent pain, weakness, or tiredness in legs when walking
Limb warmth	Limb coolness
Shortness of breath (?PE)	Ankle/foot ulceration/wounds that won't heal.
Recurrent ankle/calf swelling (SX of venous insufficiency)	Foot pain at rest

EXAM PROTOCOLS

ANKLE TO BRACHIAL INDEX (ABI)

ABIs will be performed as the basis for all protocols and options in this chapter.

The following protocol is based on recommendations by the American Heart Association: Measurement and Interpretation of the Ankle-Brachial Index : A Scientific Statement From the American Heart Association published in 2012.[3] Much of the protocol is adapted from the report.

- The patient should be in a basal state, at rest for 5 to 10 minutes in the supine position. The head and heels should be supported (not hanging over the edge of the bed). Testing should be performed in a warm room. (This period can be used for obtaining the patient history and physical)

- The patient should not smoke at least 1-2 hours before the exam.
- Wrap both arms and both ankles with blood pressure cuffs.

Scan this QR code with a code reader App on a smartphone, iPhone or tablet to view a live demo of cuff wrap methods.

- The cuff width should be at least 40% of the limb circumference.
  - ⇒ A 10 cm wide cuff can be used at the ankles and for some arms, but it's better to go large, *if the cuff fits lengthwise.* A 12 cm wide cuff will fill the above requirement on most adults.
  - ⇒ If the cuff is too small (in width) for the girth of the limb, the pressure will be artificially high.
  - ⇒ The cuff should not be applied over a distal bypass (risk of thrombosis). Also, any open lesion posing potential contamination should be covered with an impermeable dressing (Tegaderm, or clear plastic wrap (Saran Wrap) works well).
- The ankle cuffs should be 1-2 cm superior to the medial malleolus, *and wrapped snugly* (this takes practice).
- The 8 - 10 MHz CW Doppler transducer (probe) is placed over the right brachial artery or the radial artery (much easier) at a 45-60° angle to the skin. Use plenty of acoustic gel. Move the probe across the artery to maximize the signal. Appropriate method is illustrated in the Instrumentation chapter.

- Hold the Doppler probe close to the crystal end, as though you were using it as a writing utensil.
- The cuff should be inflated up to 20 mmHg above the level of flow signal disappearance and then deflated slowly to detect the flow signal reappearance. Note and record the returning systolic pressure.
  - ⇒ The maximum inflation is 300 mm Hg; if the flow is still detected, the cuff should be deflated rapidly to avoid patient discomfort.
  - ⇒ Try to avoid the common errors discussed in the Instrumentation chapter, i.e., probe sliding off the artery in supra-systolic phase, or inadvertent compression of the artery by excessive probe pressure.

> The next step, advocated by the consensus panel of the AHA, is contrary to most published protocols, and differs from the sequence employed by many manufactures, BUT, it makes sense. The recommended sequence is right arm, right PTA, right DPA, left PTA, left DPA, left arm, and repeat on right arm.

- Proceed to the right PTA. Position the Doppler probe posterior to the medial malleolus (towards the Achilles tendon, but not inferior. (You're more likely to get a reliable, consistent result if you're sitting down, and well-positioned when acquiring the ankle pressures).

CW Doppler on posterior tibial artery

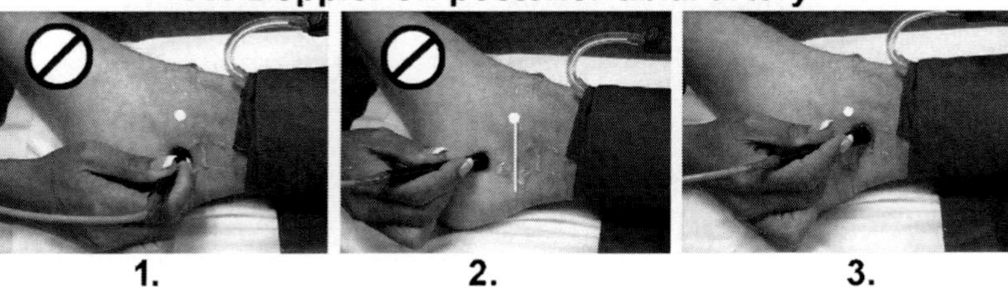

Image #1: the Doppler probe is positioned over the artery at a 90° angle; this is not good.

Image #2: The Doppler probe is positioned to far distal to the medial malleolus (the dot on the ankle marks the center of the MM). The probe is over the location of the smaller plantar artery. Try to keep the probe forward of the line on the image.

Image #3: Probe is in a good position over the PTA with a good angle (45-60°) and pointed parallel to the long axis of the artery. On most patients you can press the probe into the skin over the PTA without compressing the artery. This helps to stabilize the probe and reduce slippage.

Tip: On most patients you can gently press the probe into the skin over the PTA without compressing the artery. This helps to stabilize the probe and reduce slippage.

Scan this QR code with a code reader App on a smartphone, iPhone or tablet to view a live demo of Doppler transducer positioning methods.

- Obtain the PTA pressure as described above. Remember to optimize the Doppler signal before starting cuff inflation
- Try to gauge the inflation pressure based on the brachial pressure, particularly on automated systems where the "target" pressure can be set.
  - ⇒ For example, if the brachial pressure is 100 mmHg, initially inflate the ankle cuff to 140 or 150 mmHg. If you inflate to 200 mmHg, there will be a very long "bleed down" time until the pulse returns; you're more likely to slide off the artery location (the most common error).
  - ⇒ If the brachial pressure is high, e.g., 210 mmHg, then your inflation target pressure must be significantly higher, perhaps 250 mmHg.
  - ⇒ If the inflation system is manual and you have control

over graduated inflation pressure, inflate to 20-30 mmHg above the pressure where the Doppler signal disappeared, then start bleed-down.

⇒ In some patients the tibial arteries cannot be occluded due to calcific medial sclerosis. *In automated systems make sure that the correct cuff is inflating, i.e., the same side where your Doppler is held. If you keep increasing the pressure in the left cuff, but you're monitoring the right PTA, you won't be able to occlude the right artery no matter how high you've pumped the pressure!!*

- After the right PTA, obtain other pressures (in the following sequence): right DPA, left PTA, left DPA, left arm, *then repeat right arm.*

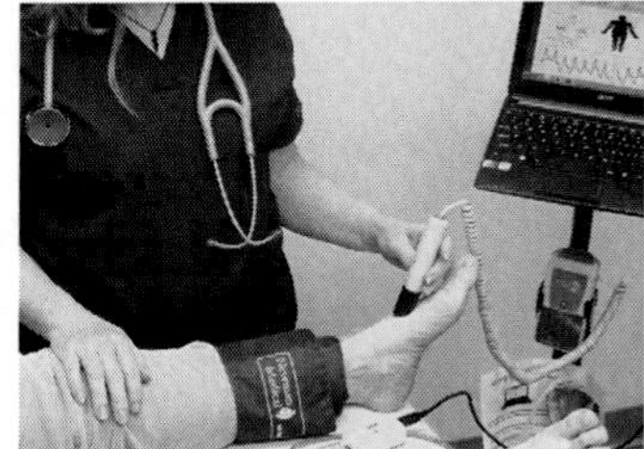

Doppler on DPA

- Pedal pressures commonly need to be repeated to resolve ambiguity or inconsistency.

> Due to extensive collateral pathways in the foot and ankle, the PTA and DPA pressures should be within 15% of each other (exceptions exist with distal bypass grafts). If the ankle pressures on the same limb are divergent by more than this amount, it's probably a technical error; so repeat each measurement.

- If the difference between the 2 right arm measurements exceeds 10 mmHg, the first measurement should be disregarded and only the second measurement used.[3]

⇒ The second right arm measurement is used to temper the effect of patient anxiety that may increase systemic pressure when the exam begins, i.e., the "white coat" effect.

⇒ Using the higher of the 2 right arm pressures is a moot point if the left arm is higher, as the higher of the brachial measurements is used for ABI calculation.

- A pressure gradient between the right and left arm of 20 mmHg or greater suggests subclavian disease on the lower side. Some reports suggest a gradient of 15 mmHg or greater is significant.[4] This finding should be confirmed with pulse volume recording, Doppler waveform analysis, or duplex imaging.
- The ABI of each leg should be calculated by dividing the higher of the PTA or DPA pressure by the higher of the right or left arm systolic blood pressure.
- For detecting PAD, the higher of the 2 ABIs for each leg should be reported.
- When ABI is used as a prognostic marker of cardiovascular events and mortality, a single ABI should be reported; report the lower of the ABIs of the left or right leg. [5]

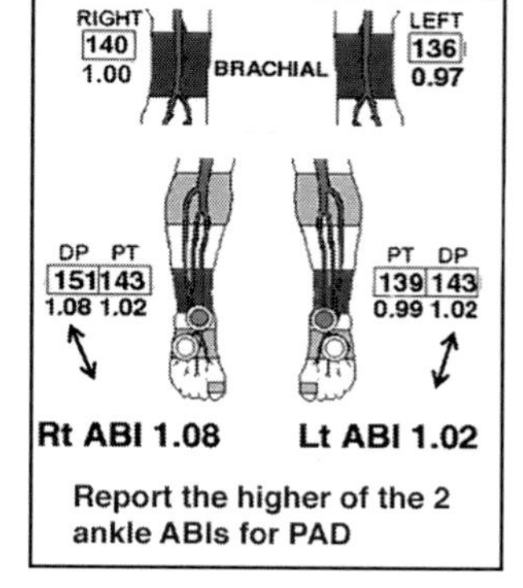

⇒ Individuals with ABI < 0.90 were twice as likely to have prevalent coronary heart disease (CHD).[6]

⇒ The chance of cardiovascular mortality significantly increases in an individual with an ABI < 0.90. [7]

Resting ABI Values

> 1.40 = probable calcified arteries.

0.90 - 1.39 = normal

< 0.90 = abnormal, perform stress test, if appropriate.

< 0.80 = probable claudication.

< 0.50 = multi-segment disease or long segment occlusion.

≤ 0.30 = ischemic rest pain, severe disease

NOTE: If brachial systolic pressure is below 100 mmHg or above 200 mmHg, ankle pressures may be 25 % lower than brachial pressure in an otherwise normal patient.[8]

Calcified Arteries: The "Bane" of Pressure Measurements:

Calcific medial sclerosis is a significant limitation for ankle pressures and ABIs. Calcium deposits in the arterial wall stiffen the wall to a point where it's incompressible. Cuff pressure cannot obliterate the distal arterial pulse so that pressure recordings are unobtainable, or are erroneously high. This condition can occur in patients with diabetes, end-stage renal disease and those on long-term corticosteroid therapy.

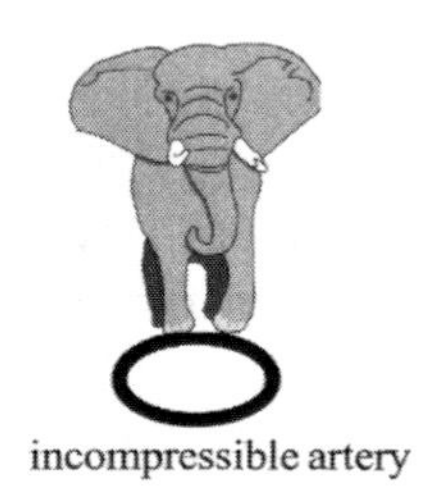
incompressible artery

You can rely on a low pressure recording, but not a high one. In the presence of calcific medial sclerosis and incompressible vessels, limb perfusion must be assessed with other methods, e.g., PVR, Doppler waveform analysis, or toe pressures. These will be discussed later in this chapter.

In general, the ankle cuff should be inflated to a pressure 30-40 mmHg above brachial pressure and “bled down”. In hypertensive patients, the increased inflation pressure required to stop flow should not be misinterpreted as calcified vessels.

Other clues to calcified arteries include:

⇒ An ABI exceeding 1.35 [9]

⇒ High closing pressure (cessation of Doppler signal during inflation) with low opening pressure.

CMS/Medicare and Noninvasive Physiologic Testing

The Center for Medicare & Medicaid Services (CMS) has established standard rules and guidelines for using physiologic studies to detect PAD.

There are a few CMS/Medicare statements worth mentioning.

⇒ "An ABI (1) is not a reimbursable procedure in itself, and (2) should be abnormal (e.g., < 0.9 at rest) or must be accompanied by another appropriate indication before proceeding to more sophisticated or complete studies, except in patients with severe diabetes resulting in medical calcification as demonstrated by artifactually elevated ankle blood pressures".[10]

⇒ "Noninvasive physiologic studies are performed using equipment separate and distinct from the duplex ultrasound imager".[10] This means you cannot use a duplex ultrasound system to acquire Doppler waveforms or pressures in any of the physiologic studies (93922, 93923, 93924).

The following are indications listed in the LCD for Novitas-Solutions, a Medicare contractor. Most Medicare contractors have similar statements. The indications below apply to physiologic testing and duplex imaging.

Indications for Peripheral Arterial Evaluations [10]

a. Claudication of less than one block or of such severity that it interferes significantly with the patient's occupation or lifestyle.

b. Rest pain (typically including the forefoot) usually associated with absent pulses, which becomes increasingly severe with elevation and diminishes with placement of the leg in a dependent position.

c. Tissue loss defined as gangrene, pre-gangrenous changes of the extremity, or ischemic ulceration of the extremity occurring in the absence of pulses.

d.. Aneurysmal disease.

e. Evidence of thromboembolic events.

f. Blunt or penetrating trauma (including complications of diagnostic and/or therapeutic procedures).

g. For evaluation of dialysis access, see policy regarding 93990.

h. Evaluation of therapeutic outcome.

i. Signs of vascular compromise include all of the following:
   - Symptoms in the extremity;
   - Past medical history; and abnormal findings on physical exam.

j. Evaluation of suspected vascular & perivascular abnormalities, including such entities as masses, aneurysms, pseudoaneurysms, or various communications between arteries and veins

The protocols below are based on the 3 Current Procedural Terminology (CPT®) codes issues for noninvasive physiologic arterial testing.

LIMITED, BILATERAL PHYSIOLOGIC STUDY

Limited, bilateral noninvasive physiologic studies of upper or lower extremity arteries (CPT code 93922)

There are 3 options for this code; the third option, $TCPO_2$, will not be discussed, as it's an uncommon test modality used primarily to determine limb amputation level. Patient preparation applies to all options.

Patient Preparation

- Greet the patient, introduce yourself, and explain the examination.
- All pressures are measured with the patient supine and in a warm room. The patient should be supine for 5–10 minutes prior to obtaining pressures to ensure a basal state.
- Obtain a history and physical as detailed earlier in the chapter in ABI Protocol.

- Apply pressure cuffs snugly to the arms and legs during this period (see QR code on page 37). The feet and ankles should be supported and not hanging over the edge of the bed.

Limited, bilateral noninvasive physiologic study

Option 1

Patient prep as discussed.

Obtain ABIs from the PTA and DPA bilaterally, as described above in the ABI protocol. Acquire pulse volume recordings (PVR, aka VPR) from the ankles, bilaterally.

- The same cuffs for blood pressures are used for PVRs. The cuffs must be uniformly wrapped and snug,
- Use 10 or 12 cm wide cuffs.
- Cuffs are connected to the plethysmograph and inflated to a specific air pressure (65 ± 5 mmHg).
  - ⇒ Some manufacturers list the volume of air injected into each cuff for contralateral comparison. Amplitude differences can occur if cuffs are asymmetrically snug and there is a significant volume difference.
- Instruct the patient to be still and silent during the test to minimize motion artifact in the tracing (it may take a few moments for the PVR waveforms to stabilize).
- Set the PVR gain to optimize the waveform amplitude, but use the same gain setting on both sides..
- PVR waveforms are then recorded for each ankle segment.
- Although a full sweep containing 3-5 waveforms is desired, only one or two good waveforms are necessary for diagnosis.

> TIP. Many elderly patients have a slight tremor in their limbs and this adversely affects the PVR waveforms. If motion artifact is present in the waveform, have the patient perform a few plantar-flexions, followed by a few moments of relaxation, then re-record the PVRs. Often this will momentarily eliminate the artifact. The technique works with PVRs at the calf, and metatarsal sites as well.

The PVR waveforms are combined with the ABI in the report page.

You also have the option of acquiring both PVRs and Doppler waveforms. This is useful when the PVR waveforms are of poor quality and are non-diagnostic.

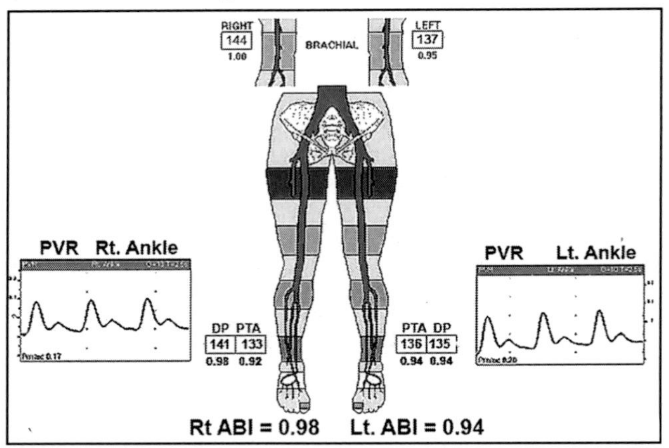

Normal, limited, bilateral physiologic study with PVRs.

- PVRs can also be obtained from the metatarsal and great toe sites if small vessel disease is suspected.
  - ⇒ Cuff sizes (bladder width) are: metatarsal (6–8 cm), great toe (2.0–2.5 cm).
  - ⇒ The metatarsal and great toe PVRs usually require a higher gain setting, as the tissue volume contained within these cuffs is obviously less than other cuff segments.

- Optionally, great toe pressures can be obtained in both options 1 and 2, and a toe/brachial index (TBI) calculated.

Limited, bilateral noninvasive physiologic study

Option 2

Obtain ABIs from the PTA and DPA bilaterally, as described above in the ABI protocol. Acquire bidirectional CW Doppler waveforms from both PTA and DPA bilaterally.

- Using good transducer technique (described in Instrumentation chapter and in the ABI section), obtain and record waveforms from the right PTA and DPA, then the left PTA and DPA.
    - ⇒ It's not unusual to find a dominate tibial vessel, usually the PTA, with a strong Doppler signal, and then find a weak DPA signal. This is most likely due to differences in vessel size and flow volume.
- Optimize the Doppler gain or scale, and use the same gain/ scale for the contralateral sites.
- The Doppler waveforms are combined with the ABI in the report page.

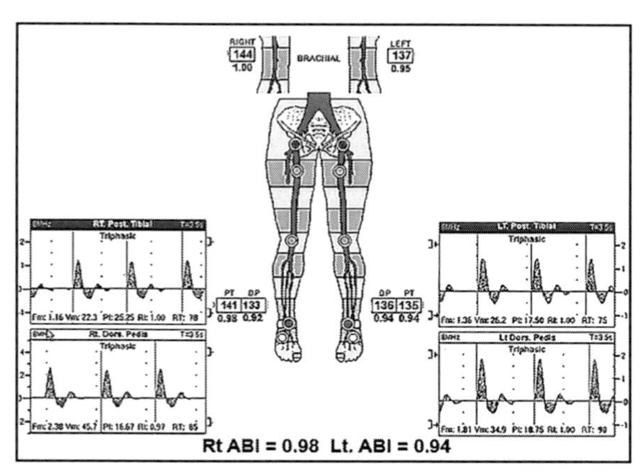

Normal, limited, bilateral physiologic study with Doppler spectral waveforms.

COMPLETE, BILATERAL PHYSIOLOGIC STUDY

Complete bilateral noninvasive physiologic studies of upper or lower extremity arteries at <u>3 or more levels</u> (CPT 93923)

As the description indicates, this test is an extension of the limited study, and includes calf and thigh test sites. There are options in the CPT description for the multi-level exam. One option involves segmental Doppler waveforms and pressures, the other with segmental PVR waveforms.

Complete Bilateral Study

<u>Option 1</u>

Option 1 includes ABI with segmental PVR waveforms from the ankle, calf, and thigh levels, bilaterally. Metatarsal and great toe PVRs can be obtained as needed, as well as a great toe pressure for a toe/brachial index.

Pressure Cuff Application for PVRs

With the patient in a supine position with the heel of the foot placed upon a pillow or pad, apply blood pressure cuffs to the following locations. The cuffs should be appropriately sized (see below) and be applied very snugly; fingers should slide between cuff and limb with difficulty. All cuff sizes refer to the cuff air bladder width.

⇒ Upper arms (10 or 12 cm).

⇒ Upper thighs (12 cm).

⇒ Lower thighs (12 cm).

⇒ Proximal calves (AKA, below knee) (12 cm).

⇒ Ankles (10 or 12 cm).

⇒ Optional: metatarsals (6–8 cm), great toes (2.0–2.5 cm).

- The low-thigh cuff (4-cuff technique) should be positioned against the upper cuff, and should not extend over the knee. If two cuffs will not fit on the thigh, use only one 12 cm cuff positioned high on the thigh. Alternatively, use one 17 cm-wide cuff.
- Obtain ankle to brachial indices as described earlier in this chapter. Use the AHA recommended sequence: right arm, right PTA & DPA, left PTA & DPA, left arm, then repeat right arm.

Pulse Volume Recording

- The sequence of PVR acquisition sites is often dictated by system software; either thigh, calf, ankle, or ankle, calf, thigh. Manual override is available, so any site can be selected. Most systems allow simultaneous, bilateral acquisition.
- Cuffs are sequentially connected to the plethysmograph and inflated to a specific air pressure (65 ± 5 mmHg).
- Some manufacturers list the volume of air injected into each cuff for contralateral comparison. Amplitude differences can occur if there is a significant volume discrepancy from side to side.
- Instruct the patient to be still and silent during the test to minimize motion artifact in the tracing.
- Set the PVR gain to optimize the waveform amplitude, but use the same gain setting on both sides.
  - ⇒ Some labs will obtain PVRs at the calf level first, so they can optimize and standardize the gain at that level. The calf usually has the highest PVR amplitude (in normals), so this gain setting works well for the thigh and ankle sites.
- PVR waveforms are then recorded for each segment.

- Although a full sweep containing 3-5 waveforms is desired, only one or two waveforms are necessary for a diagnosis.

Helpful hints on cuff application

- Do not let the patient lift their leg in an attempt to assist you when applying thigh or calf cuffs; as soon as they relax their muscles, the cuffs become loose.
- In the legs, start the cuff wrap with the bladder on the posterior-medial aspect of the limb, bring the cuff one full wrap, then pull upward and across to tighten the wrap; try not to get your hand caught in the folds of the cuff!
- Place the upper thigh cuff as proximal as possible.
- The low-thigh cuff (4-cuff technique) should be positioned against the upper cuff, and should not extend over the knee. If two cuffs will not fit on the thigh, use only one 12 cm cuff positioned high on the thigh. Alternatively, use a wide 17 cm thigh cuff.
- Cuffs may be placed over thin clothing, for example, hospital pajamas etc., as pressures or PVRs will not be affected.

Interpretation

⇒ Pulse waveform analysis is a qualitative assessment (pattern recognition) of pulse contour and amplitude. It is a subjective assessment of overall limb perfusion.

⇒ If the thigh PVR is normal, there is no significant inflow (aortoiliac) disease.

⇒ Pulse volume waveforms reflect the volume of blood coming into that cuff segment; so an abnormal PVR at the thigh would indicate aortoiliac disease, or more rarely, profunda femoris artery stenosis.

⇒ *Volume changes in the thigh cuff are predominately*

affected by perfusion in the deep femoral system.

⇒ If the thigh PVR is normal, but the calf is abnormal, the occlusive disease will be in the superficial femoral and/or popliteal segments.

⇒ Proximal disease will affect the contour of all PVRs distally.

⇒ PVR amplitude in the calf may be higher than the amplitude of the thigh and ankle (particularly with the 3-cuff method). This is due to variations in limb girth, cuff size and air volume within the cuff.

⇒ Normal thigh and calf PVRs with abnormal ankle PVRs suggests tibial disease.

⇒ PVRs are not affected by calcified arteries and are easier to perform than CW Doppler waveform analysis.

A normal PVR waveform has a sharp upslope and a prominent reflected wave in late systole and early diastole.

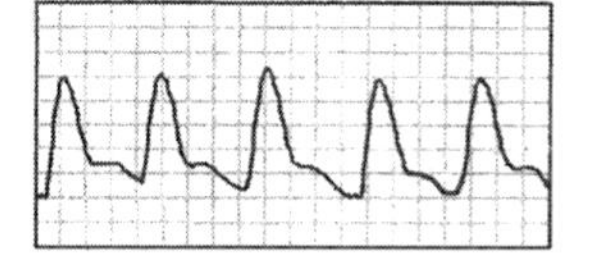

Mild disease will cause the waveform to broaden and the reflected wave (dicrotic notch) will not be present. There is also a slight loss of amplitude.

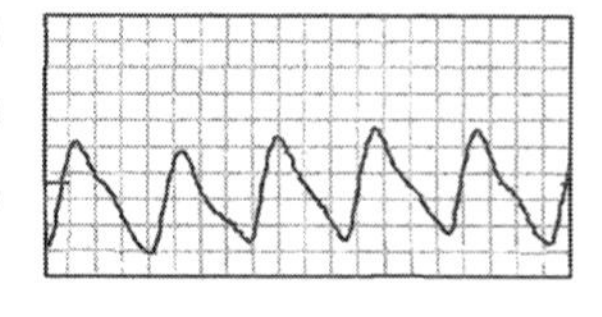

A moderately abnormal PVR has a rounded peak, no reflected wave and a pronounced decrease in amplitude.

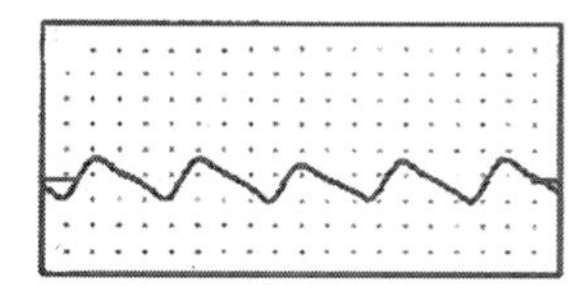

A severely abnormal PVR is of low amplitude, or even "flatline".

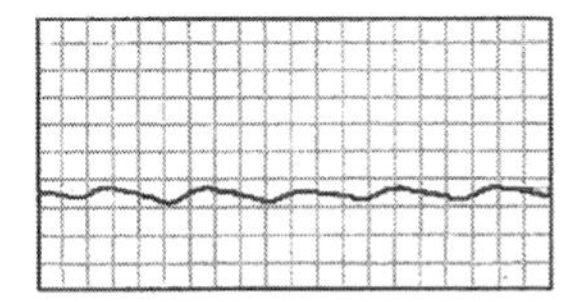

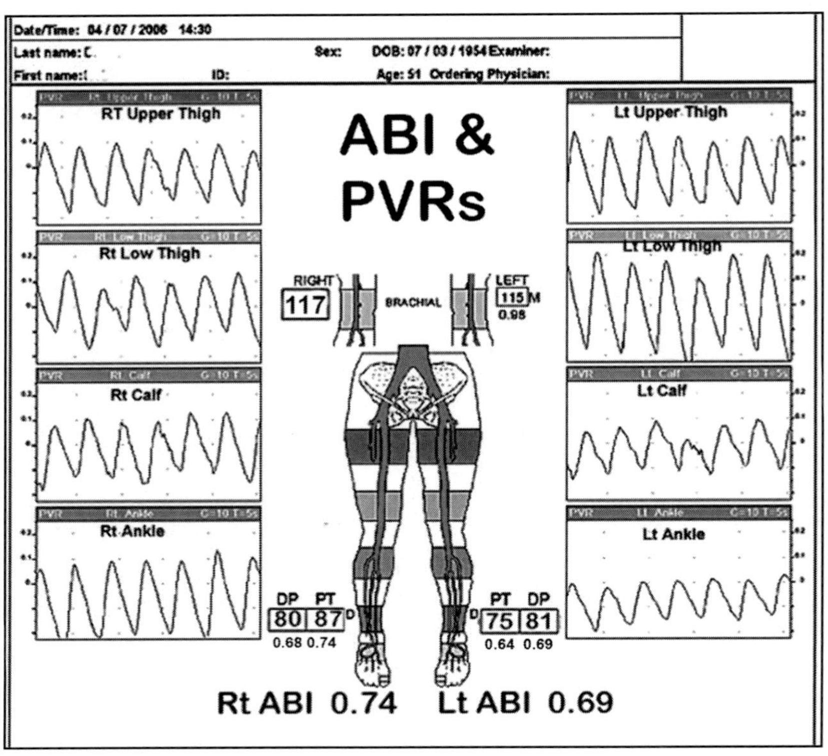

ABIs are abnormal bilaterally. The PVR waveforms are abnormal at the upper thigh level, bilaterally. This indicates moderate inflow (aortoiliac) disease. Note; thigh pressures were not necessary to make this diagnosis.

Complete Bilateral Study

Option 2

ABIs (from both PTA & DPA bilaterally) plus segmental blood pressure measurements with bidirectional Doppler waveform recording and analysis, at 3 or more levels.

This protocol is more complex, and involves segmental pressure determination at multiple levels, as well as segmental Doppler waveform analysis.

Segmental Pressure Sequence Options

The traditional sequence for segmental pressures is right arm, left arm, right DPA and PTA. The Doppler probe remains over the PTA for the subsequent calf, low-thigh, and high-thigh pressures. The sequence is then repeated on the left leg.

This method is convenient, as once the PTA pressure is obtained, the transducer does not have to be moved or relocated for the calf and thigh pressures for that leg. Unfortunately, this method is not in accord with the sequence recommended by the American Heart Association (AHA) for ABI.[3] The AHA, to my knowledge, has not recommended a sequence for segmental limb pressures.

To use the AHA method with segmental pressures: obtain pressures in the following order (as described in the ABI protocol): Rt. arm, Rt. PTA, Rt. DPA. Lt. PTA, Lt. DPA, Lt. arm, Rt. arm (repeated). Then return to the PTA, acquire an optimum signal, and obtain Rt. calf, low-thigh and high-thigh pressures. Move to the left PTA and acquire the Lt. calf, low-thigh, and high-thigh pressures of that leg.

The methods described below are the traditional segmental pressure sequence.

Pressure Cuff Application

- Apply cuffs to arms and legs as described in Complete Bilateral Study, Option 1.
- Place the calf (below knee) cuff below the bony structures of the knee, otherwise, excessively high pressures may be recorded.

Three–cuff versus Four–cuff methods

- There are two methods for full segmental pressure testing: the three-cuff and the four-cuff methods.

- The *three-cuff* method uses one large (17 cm air bladder) thigh cuff, plus calf and ankle cuffs.
- The large thigh cuff is contoured and fits the thigh better than a non-contoured 12 cm cuff.
- Most automated cuff inflation systems use a 4-cuff method, as the air pump capacity is inadequate for the large air volume necessary to inflate the 17 cm cuff.

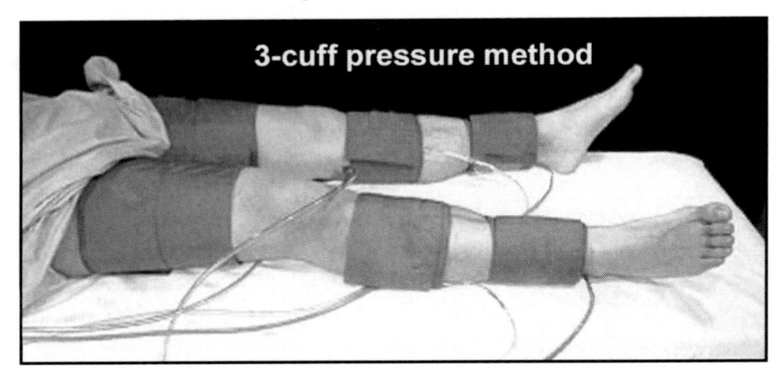

- The *four-cuff* method uses two smaller thigh cuffs (12 cm), as well as 2 cuffs below the knee. With segmental pressures, the four-cuff method is reported to be better at differentiating inflow disease from femoral artery disease.[11]

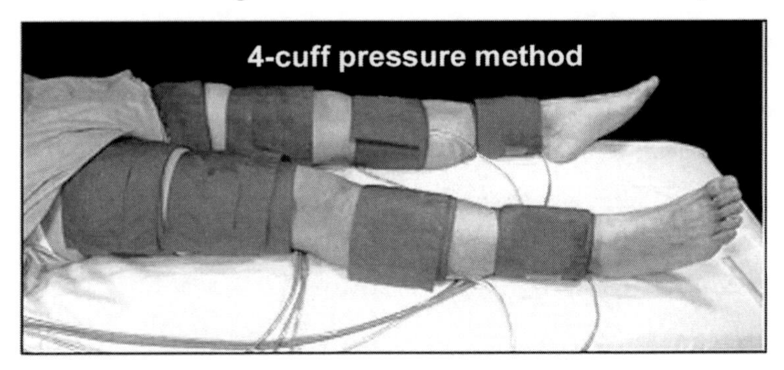

- The low-thigh cuff (4-cuff technique) should be positioned against the upper cuff, and should not extend over the knee. If two cuffs will not fit on the thigh, use only one 12 cm cuff positioned high on the thigh.

See Helpful hints on cuff application described in option 1

Segmental Pressures

Bilateral arm pressures

- Place a CW Doppler over the radial (preferred method) or the brachial artery and locate the strongest signal by sweeping across the entire artery, then back to the center.
- Inflate the cuff manually, or with auto-inflation device, until the signal is obliterated, continue increasing pressure for an additional 15 or 20 mmHg. Slowly bleed the pressure down until the signal returns, and mark or note the return pressure from the pressure manometer or digital display. Stop the sequence (freeze) and rapidly deflate the cuff pressure to zero.
  - ⇒ If possible, allow a few "beats" to be recorded on the Doppler display after the initial return pulse. This helps to verify that it is indeed a pulse reappearance and not random noise.
- Repeat pressure if any ambiguity or inconsistency occurs.
- Obtain systolic pressure in the right arm, then the left arm.
- Use the higher of the two arm pressures for subsequent leg comparisons and for calculating ABI.
- ***Do not obtain a blood pressure in an arm with a shunt or dialysis access graft.***

Try to avoid the 2 most common errors; the transducer sliding off the artery, and inadvertent compression of the artery underneath the probe. Mistakes are bound to occur; the trick is knowing when you've made a technical error.

Obtain ankle and other limb pressures

- Place the Doppler probe over the right DPA on top of the foot, optimize the signal and inflate the ankle cuff. With the methods described above, obtain the DPA pressure.
- Place the Doppler probe over the right PTA, inflate the ankle cuff and obtain the PTA pressure.

Calf Level

- With the transducer still over the right PTA, inflate the calf cuff while monitoring blood flow at the ankle and obtain calf pressure.
  - ⇒ The measured pressure at each cuff level is the pressure in the artery segment under the cuff, regardless of where the Doppler is held.

> TIP: If calf and thigh pressures are to be obtained, experienced technologists prefer to use the PTA as the monitoring vessel, as pressure errors (inadvertent compression, probe drift, etc.) are less likely to occur with this artery than with the DPA.

Thigh Level

- With both the single, large cuff (3-cuff technique) and the 12 cm cuff (4-cuff technique), the cuffs should be wrapped tightly, and positioned as high as possible on the thigh. A loosely wrapped cuff takes a very long (*painful*) time to reach appropriate inflation levels.
- Instruct the patient that this pressure measurement may be uncomfortable and caution him/her not to move the leg during the test.
- While monitoring flow at the PTA, quickly inflate the thigh cuff to suprasystolic levels and then bleed back down.

- Many patients cannot tolerate the discomfort and pain of thigh pressure, especially if they're hypertensive and the cuff must be inflated to very high level. If thigh pressures are necessary, they should be performed quickly and precisely. Get it right the first time!
- Short Cut: If the ankle and calf pressures are normal (eg.,normal ABI), **skip the thigh pressure measurements**, as they'll be normal as well.
- The high-thigh cuff (12 cm size) usually must be inflated to 40 mmHg above the arm pressure.
- Because the high-thigh cuff is narrow compared to limb girth, **a pressure artifact** usually (but not always) exists that elevates the pressure value 20 - 30 mmHg above systemic pressure or the true intra-arterial pressure. It's called the **high-thigh cuff artifact**

Toe Pressures (optional)

- Toe pressures are useful in evaluating small vessel disease and in diabetic patients with calcified, incompressible tibial arteries. Toe pressures are difficult to obtain in patients with small vessel disease, as perfusion may be severely compromised. In most circumstances however, toe pressure is an optional test when ankle pressures are normal.
- Pressures are obtained by placing a small (1.9 or 2.5 cm) digital cuff on the great toe and recording systolic pressure with a PPG transducer positioned distally on the toe.
- PPG waveforms must be present for toe pressures; if PPG waveforms are flat line, pressures cannot be obtained.
- Obtain baseline PPG pulses on the toe, adjust the scale or gain, and inflate the cuff(s) until waveforms are obliterated. Bleed pressure back down slowly until the PPG pulsatile trace returns. Align the measurement caliper with the first

"real" pulse (don't measure a noise artifact) and obtain the toe systolic pressure.

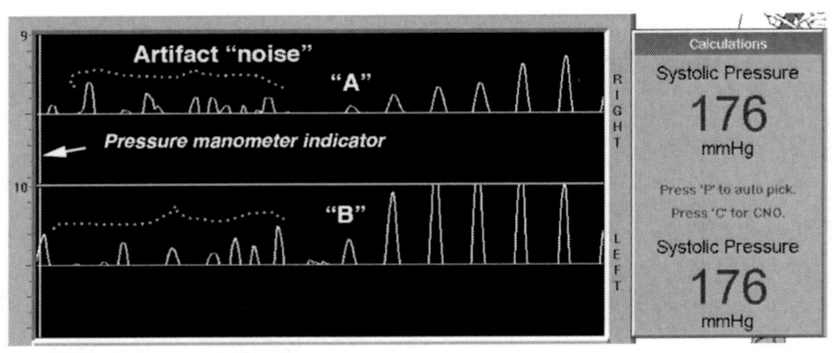

This is an example of a bad toe pressure test. There is excessive "noise" artifact in the PPG trace. The system automatically aligned the measurement cursor (vertical white line) with the first "blips" and these are not the returning pressure pulse. The pressure is incorrectly registered at 176 mmHg bilaterally. The operator should have positioned the measurements cursors at point A and B. Or better, repeated the test with reduced noise artifact.

- Noise artifact can be caused by motion adjacent to the PPG transducers, excessive gain, and by toe movement. Light interference can also cause a reaction in the PPG sensors. If light interference is suspected, cover the toe and PPG with a dark towel.
- Pressures can be obtained with Doppler as well, but it's more difficult, as the digit arterial signal is hard to locate. It's also difficult to obtain pressures on the 4 smaller toes, and they're probably inaccurate due to the size of the toe compared to the cuff size.
- A Toe/Brachial Index may be calculated by dividing each toe pressure by the higher brachial pressure. There is wide variation of TBI values in the literature, but a TBI of less than 0.60 can be considered abnormal.[12]

Doppler Waveform Analysis

Continuous-wave (CW), bi-directional Doppler waveforms are obtained and recorded at specific sites along the major arteries in each leg in "option 2" of the **complete bilateral physiologic study**. Waveforms are subjectively assessed and compared to adjacent and contralateral sites for abnormality.

As described in Chapter 2- Instrumentation, CW-Doppler waveforms are created with either zero-crossing detection method (most common) or Fast Fourier Transform spectral analysis.

Procedure

- Remove pressure cuffs for access to the sample sites.
- With the patient in a supine position and in a basal state at rest, a CW Doppler probe is positioned at a 45-60 degree angle over the common femoral artery (CFA) just below the groin crease, and pointed cephalad (towards the head). Use a lower frequency Doppler transducer, 4 or 5 MHz.
- Eliminate any intruding venous signals and try to achieve the strongest arterial signal possible.
- Record Doppler waveforms with appropriate gain settings to allow a good waveform amplitude. Use the same gain/scale setting when obtaining the waveforms from the contralateral site.

In addition to the CFA site, obtain Doppler waveforms at the following locations,bilaterally:

- ♦ Proximal and distal superficial femoral artery
- ♦ Popliteal artery
- ♦ Posterior tibial artery
- ♦ Dorsalis pedis artery

For the pedal vessels use a high frequency transducer, 8 -10 MHz.

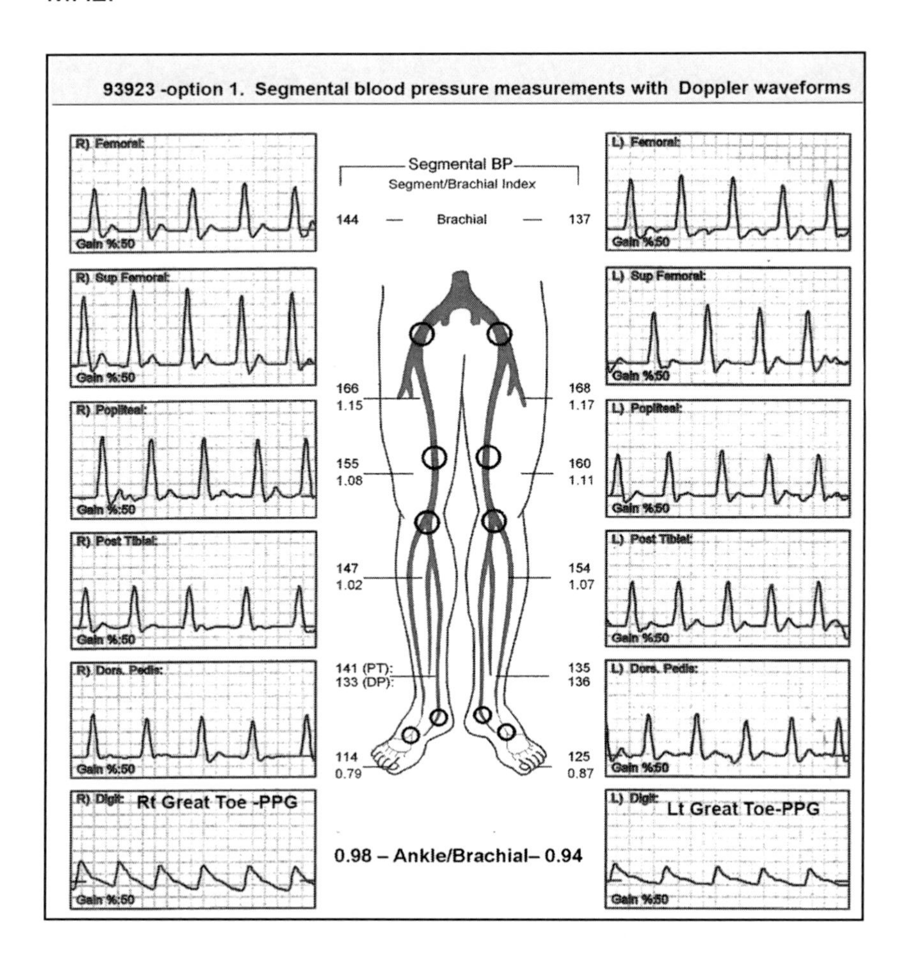

Segmental Limb Pressure Interpretation

Arm pressures:

A gradient of 15-20 mmHg or more between brachial pressures indicates subclavian stenosis/occlusion on the side of the lower pressure.[4] This finding should be confirmed with pulse volume recording, Doppler waveform analysis, or duplex imaging.

Leg pressures:

If ankle pressures and ABIs are normal, (and there is no suspicion on calcified tibial vessels), segmental limb pressures should also be normal; if they're not it's probably due to technical error or cuff artifact. For example, if a thigh pressure is low and the distal pressure is high, it's probably an error,

> NOTE: Segmental pressure gradients, in the presence of a NORMAL ABI, should not be interpreted as evidence for occlusive disease. If the ABI is normal, segmental pressure differences are "moot" for that limb.

- If ABIs are abnormal, limb pressure gradients can help locate the region of disease. Some laboratories rely on segmental waveforms, instead of segmental pressures, to determine the level of disease in the presence of an abnormal ABI.
- If ABIs are abnormal, but ankle Doppler or PVRs appear normal, recheck the pressures, as these 2 sets of data should agree.
- Thigh pressure interpretation varies depending on whether the 3-cuff or 4-cuff method was used.

Segmental Three-Cuff Technique:

Normal:

⇒ All segmental pressures, including the thigh pressure, should be equal to or slightly greater than the brachial pressure.

Abnormal:

⇒ A ≥ 30 mmHg drop in pressure between contiguous segments generally is considered positive for hemodynamically significant stenosis (> 60% diameter) in the segment(s) leading into the cuff or under the cuff (as long as the more proximal cuff pressure is not artificially elevated, and the ABI is abnormal).

⇒ A normal thigh pressure usually rules out significant aortoiliac disease. An abnormal thigh pressure can be due to aortoiliac disease, or femoral artery disease.[13]

Segmental Four-Cuff Technique:

Normal:

⇒ The high-thigh pressure should be at least 20 mmHg above brachial pressure due to the “high-thigh cuff artifact”.

⇒ However, variations in the girth of the thigh relative to the fixed cuff size often eliminate the cuff artifact. If the thigh is relatively small, the thigh pressure may be equal to or near brachial pressure in a otherwise normal individual.

Abnormal:

⇒ A thigh pressure that is less than the arm pressure is abnormal and suggests inflow disease.

⇒ A pressure gradient of 30 mmHg or more between the high-thigh and low-thigh is suggestive of superficial femoral disease.

⇒ Studies have shown that a normal high-thigh pressure rules out significant aortoiliac (A-I) disease, and an abnormal high-thigh pressure will predict significant A - I disease.[11]

⇒ *Other studies, however, have shown that a low high-thigh value can be due to superficial femoral artery disease and not necessarily A-I obstruction. The negative predictive value is high, but the positive predictive valve for A-I disease is low.* [13,14]

⇒ The low-thigh, calf, and ankle pressures are interpreted as in the 3-cuff technique.

As with all indirect methods, SLPs cannot distinguish stenosis from total occlusion and are not specific in determining the exact location of disease.

Thigh pressure interpretation summary

For both the 3 and 4-cuff methods:

⇒ If proximal thigh pressures are normal, there is probably no significant inflow (aortoiliac) disease. However, there is a small subset of patients that have "hidden" aortoiliac disease, i.e., not detected in a resting exam. Post-exercise testing would reveal the disease as ankle pressure is likely to drop.

⇒ If proximal thigh pressures are abnormal, waveforms should be used to help differentiate inflow disease from femoral artery disease. Either condition can cause a decrease in thigh pressure.

Other Criteria:

Ankle pressures can quantify the severity of ischemia. A pressure of 50 mmHg or less is often associated with ischemic rest pain. In non-diabetics, foot lesions are unlikely to heal if ankle pressure is less than 50 mmHg.[2]

Doppler Waveform Interpretation

Waveforms are subjectively assessed and compared to adjacent and contralateral sites for abnormality.

ANALOG DOPPLER

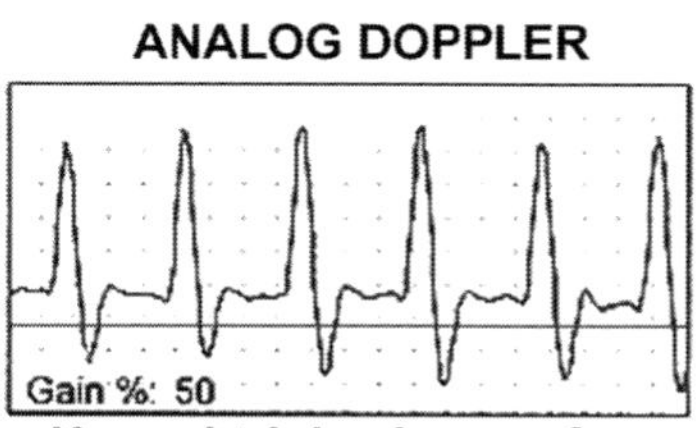

Normal triphasic waveform

SPECTRAL DOPPLER

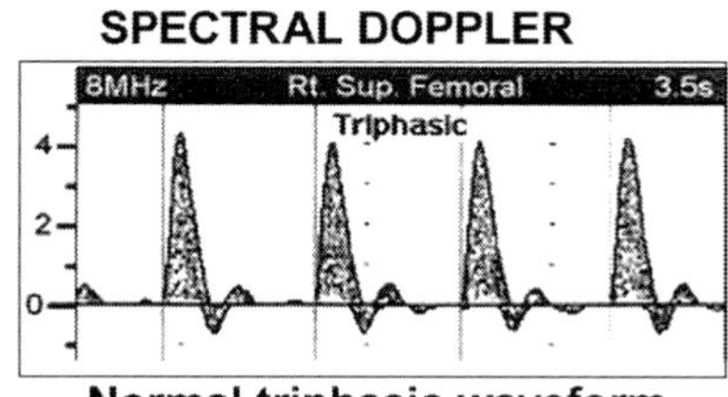

Normal triphasic waveform

- A normal waveform should be **multiphasic** with a sharp systolic upslope, an immediate drop of waveform below baseline, then a small blip of amplitude before the next systolic rise. There are a number of normal variants, and it is not uncommon to find a multiphasic waveform with the diastolic trace above baseline.
- Some normal waveforms have only a forward and a small reverse component and lack a third blip.

ANALOG DOPPLER

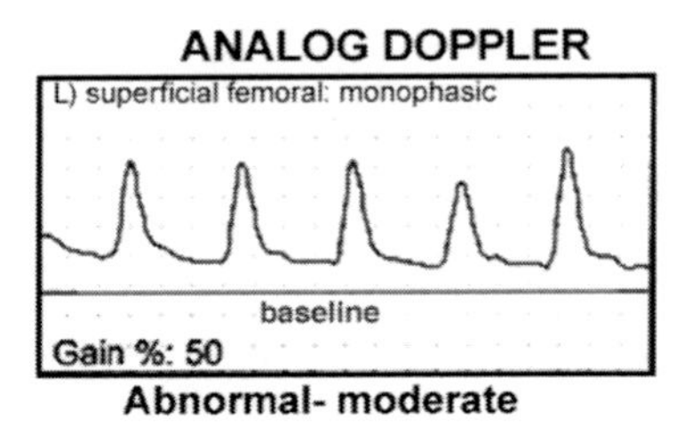

Abnormal- moderate

SPECTRAL DOPPLER

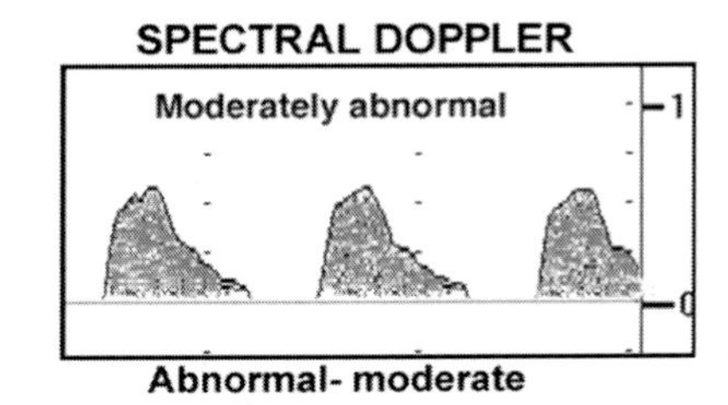

Abnormal- moderate

Moderately abnormal waveform exhibits a loss of triphasic morphology, reduced amplitude and no reverse flow component.

ANALOG DOPPLER

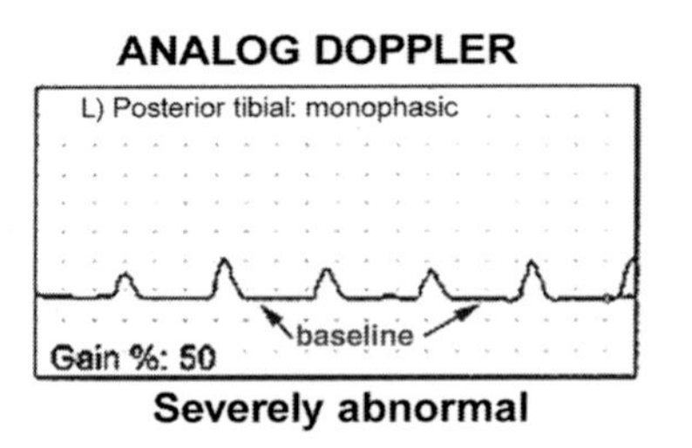

Severely abnormal

SPECTRAL DOPPLER

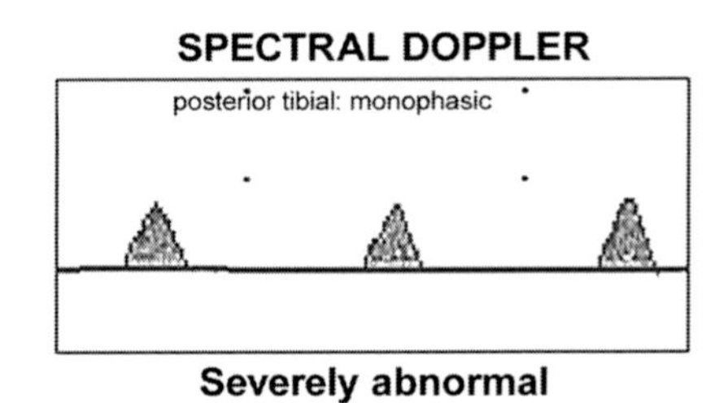

Severely abnormal

A severely abnormal Doppler waveform demonstrates an absence of triphasic pattern, loss of amplitude and delayed upstroke to peak. This is referred to as a **monophasic** waveform. Flow may be absent in diastole.

- Abnormality between segments suggests the presence of disease in that region.
- The recorded waveform must be free of artifact.
- The Doppler signal may be attenuated by obesity, scar tissue, hematoma, or calcified plaque within the artery.

- Waveform analysis is not quantitative for assessing the severity of disease, only qualitative.
- The term "biphasic" is often used to describe an abnormal peripheral arterial waveform. Because there is considerable confusion regarding what constitutes a "biphasic" waveform, the term should be abandoned and not used to describe Doppler waveform morphology; use multi-phasic, atypical-abnormal and monophasic-abnormal.
- CW Doppler technique requires skill and experience.

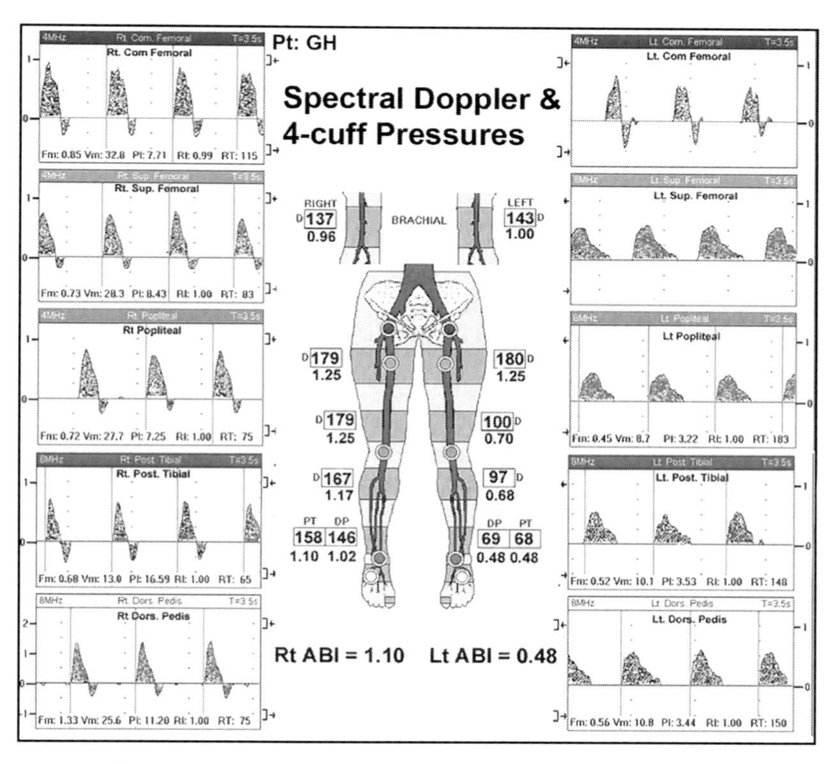

ABI is abnormal on the left. Upper thigh pressures are normal bilaterally and exhibit the high-thigh cuff artifact. There is a significant decrease in pressure at the low thigh level on the left. Doppler waveforms are normal at the CFA , and are abnormal at the left SFA and at sites below. Moderate femoro-popliteal disease on the left. Right side is normal.

Noninvasive physiologic studies of lower extremity arteries, at rest and following treadmill stress testing-CPT 93924

PHYSIOLOGIC STUDY WITH EXERCISE STRESS TESTING

- This test is important for differentiating true vascular claudication from pseudo-claudication, i.e., true ischemic muscle pain with exercise, from the pain caused by neurospinal compression, osteoarthritis, or some other non-vascular cause. Claudication-like pain with exercise that is not due to arterial obstruction is called pseudo-claudication,
- The exercise stress test is performed on a motorized treadmill on all patients that complain of pain when walking, with the exception of those that have contraindications.
- Resting blood flow over a stenotic lesion may be sufficient to maintain normal or near normal distal pressure. When flow is augmented over the stenosis, as in exercise or reactive hyperemia, distal pressure may decrease revealing the presence of disease. It is appropriate to exercise those with claudication symptoms despite a normal resting exam.
- If the patient's symptoms occur at rest (non-claudication symptoms) and the resting examination is negative, there is no need to exercise the patient.

Contraindications for Treadmill Exercise

- Questionable cardiac status, known cardio-vascular disease, or uncontrolled angina
- Severe pulmonary disease.
- Inability to ambulate at treadmill speed.
- Ischemic rest pain, or ankle pressure < 40 mmHg
- Ischemic limb ulceration.
- Non-compressible tibial arteries

> NOTE: This test does not equate to the rigors of a cardiac stress test and the risk of cardiac complications is small. It is appropriate, however, that a written protocol be established and followed in regards to exercise contraindications, methods, and response to cardiac emergency. EKG monitoring should be used if available.

Procedure

- Following the resting physiologic study, the patient is screened for contraindications. If patient has no contraindications and is a candidate, proceed.
- Explain the test to the patient, ask that they walk for 5 minutes or until the pain stops them from walking. Request that they tell you of the onset, location and severity of pain, if any. Remind them to report any chest pain, shortness of breath, or severe fatigue.
- Set treadmill speed to 1.5 or 2.0 mph at a 10% grade, depending on the patients age and mobility.
- Standard walking time is for 5 minutes or until pain or other factors (angina, SOB, fatigue, etc.) limit further walking. The patient must be carefully observed for distress during exercise and the technologist must not leave the room.
- Claudication symptoms are noted, as well as the time of onset, severity, and the total walking time. Did the claudication stop the patient, or was there some other cause?
- Immediately following exercise, return the patient to the exam bed and quickly obtain bilateral ankle pressures from either the PTA or DPA. Use the pedal artery that had the higher resting pressure. There is no need to obtain pressures from both arteries on one foot.

- Start with the ankle of the most symptomatic leg, go to the other ankle, then to the arm
- Obtain the brachial systolic pressure from the arm with the higher resting pressure.
- Post-exercise PVRs or Doppler waveforms may be useful in patients in whom pressures cannot be obtained due to calcified vessels. Pre and Post PVRs can be subjectively assessed for disease severity.
- Calculate post-exercise ABIs.

It's the opinion of this author that serial pressure acquisition following exercise is a waste of time. Color duplex imaging is a better methods to determine the extend of disease and whether there are multiple segments involved. However, changes in physiologic testing guidelines made by CMS in 2011 indicate that ABIs should be obtained at "timed intervals" following treadmill exercise, until ankle pressures have returned to pre-exercise levels.

- If the post-exercise pressures are normal and no pressure drop has occurred at the ankles, there is no need to continue with serial pressure measurements.
- If a pressure drop occurred in either ankle, repeat ABIs at 2 minute intervals until pressures return to pre-exercise levels.

A prolonged recovery time suggests multilevel disease, or poor collateralization. In the example below, the left ankle is normal, but the right ankle demonstrated significant post exercise pressure decrease with slow recovery time.

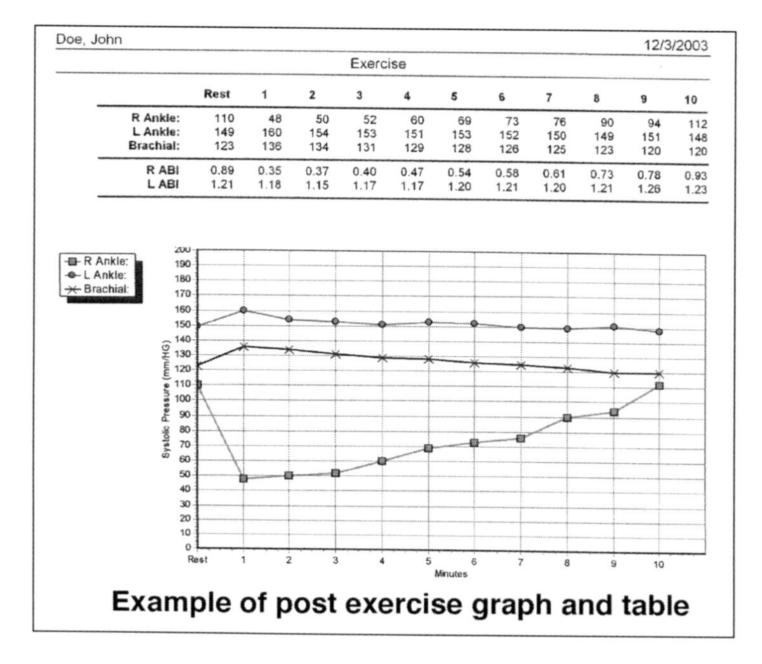

Doe, John 12/3/2003

Exercise

	Rest	1	2	3	4	5	6	7	8	9	10
R Ankle:	110	48	50	52	60	69	73	76	90	94	112
L Ankle:	149	160	154	153	151	153	152	150	149	151	148
Brachial:	123	136	134	131	129	128	126	125	123	120	120
R ABI	0.89	0.35	0.37	0.40	0.47	0.54	0.58	0.61	0.73	0.78	0.93
L ABI	1.21	1.18	1.15	1.17	1.17	1.20	1.21	1.20	1.21	1.26	1.23

Example of post exercise graph and table

Interpretation

- Some normal patients may experience a very mild, transient drop in ankle pressure following exercise, while others will maintain a normal ankle/brachial index.
- Those with arterial occlusive disease will experience a pressure drop of varying degree, depending on the severity of disease and the amount of collateral blood flow.
- A pressure decrease of > 30 mm Hg or a post-exercise ABI decrease of > 20% indicates PAD.[3]
- An immediate post-exercise ankle pressure of 60 mmHg or less confirms a vascular cause for claudication. A vascular etiology for pain is unlikely if immediate post-exercise ankle pressures are well above 60 mmHg.[2] Vascular claudication pain is a transient “ischemic” pain.
- Post-exercise pressures must be obtained as soon as possible following cessation of exercise. Ankle pressures

will rise following exercise and a delay may result in erroneously high measurements.

- The CPT description for this code (93924) does not specify whether the resting exam is a limited bilateral study or a "complete" bilateral study.

> CPT code 93924 can only be applied if motorized treadmill exercise is performed. Other forms of stress testing (toe raises, etc.) are considered "provocative maneuvers" and are covered under CPT 93923. Only one of the physiologic testing codes can be submitted.

Toe Raises (heel raises)

Toes raises (active plantar flexions, also called “heel raises”) have been advocated as a useful alternative to treadmill exercise.[15] A full or limited resting study is first obtained, then ankle cuffs are removed and the procedure explained to the patient.

Procedure

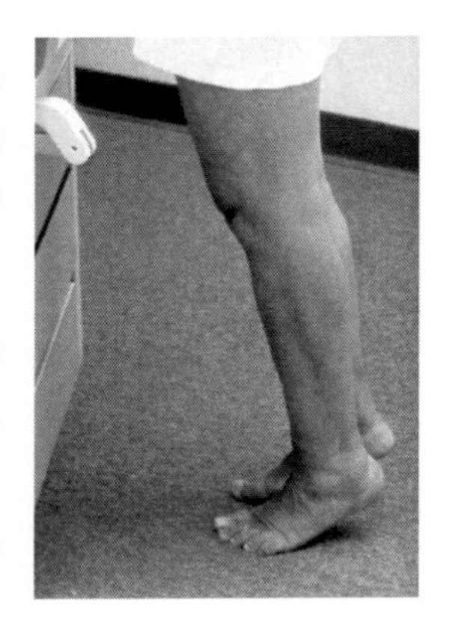

- The patient stands and extends both feet fully, then relaxes and returns the feet flat to the floor at 1 second intervals.
- The “toe raises” are repeated up to 50 times, or until the patient cannot continue.
- The onset of pain and the number of toe raises are recorded.
- Immediately after exercise, the patient returns to the exam bed and ankle/arm pressures are obtained. Obtain one brachial pressure and one ankle pressure from each leg. Use the arm and the pedal artery that had the higher resting pressure.

- Compared to the resting values; a pressure drop of >20 mmHg or a decrease in ABI of 20% constitutes an abnormal exam.[9]

Although this exercise test eliminates the need for a cumbersome treadmill and may have lower risk of cardiac complications, it does not invoke the same muscle groups used when walking, and it may not reproduce the patient's symptoms of ischemic claudication. Although the patient may have mild vascular disease and demonstrate a slight drop in pressure after toe raises, the calf pain may be solely due to fatigue. It is important to correlate claudication symptoms with a significant pressure drop to confirm a vascular etiology for the pain. This test is a substitute for treadmill stress test in patients with cardiac risk, but it is a poor substitute for treadmill exercise in patients with intermittent claudication.

It's important to remember the goals of physiologic testing, and to have appropriate expectations of what the tests can provide:

1. Is there objective evidence for PAD?
2. If disease is present, what's the severity?
3. If disease is present, is it causing the patient's symptoms?
4. If disease is present, what regions are affected?

Physiologic testing cannot provide anatomic detail, precise location of disease, or whether arteries are occluded or stenoses. It can only detect "hemodynamically significant disease, that is likely to cause symptoms.

References

1. Rutherford, RB, Lowenstein DH, Klein MF. Combining segmental systolic pressures and plethysmography to diagnose occlusive disease of the legs. Am J Surg 138:211-218, 1979
2. Raines J K, Darling R C, Bluth J., et al. Vascular laboratory criteria for the management of peripheral vascular disease of the lower extremities. Surgery 79:21, 1976

3. Aboyans V, et. al. Measurement and Interpretation of the Ankle-Brachial Index : A Scientific Statement From the American Heart Association. Circulation. 2012;126:00-00. Downloaded from http://circ.ahajourn1als.org
4. Osborn LA, Vernon SM, Reynolds B, Timm TC, Allen K. Screening for subclavian artery stenosis in patients who are candidates for coronarybypass surgery. Catheter Cardiovasc Interv. 2002;56:162–165.
5. O'Hare AM, Katz R, Shlipak MG, Cushman M, Newman AB. Mortality and cardiovascular risk across the ankle-arm index spectrum: results from the Cardiovascular Health Study. Circulation. 2006;113:388 –393.
6. Zheng ZJ Associations of ankle-brachial index with clinical coronary heart disease, stroke and preclinical carotid and popliteal atherosclerosis: the Atherosclerosis Risk in Communities (ARIC) Study. Atherosclerosis. Vol 131, issue 1, 115-125, May 1997
7. Ankle Brachial Index Collaboration, Fowkes FG, et.at. Ankle brachial index combined with Framingham risk score to predict cardiovascular events and mortality: a meta-analysis. JAMA. 2008;300:197–208.
8. Belcaro et al. Noninvasive Diagnostic Techniques in Vascular Disease. E. Bernstein, editor, third edition P 507 Mosby, St. Louis
9. Carter SA. Clinical measurement of systolic pressure in limbs with arterial occlusive disease JAMA 1969;207:1869-1874
10. Novitas Solutions LCD L32754 Non Invasive Vascular Studies. https://www.novitas-solutions.com/policy/jh/l32754-r5.html
11. Heintz SE, Bone GE, Slaymaker EE, Hayes AC, Barnes RW. Value of arterial pressure measurements in the proximal and distal part of the thigh in arterial occlusive disease. Surg Gynocol Obstet:146:337-43,1978
12. Bridges RA, Barnes RW. Segmental limb pressures. In: Kempczinski RF and Yao SJS. Practical Noninvasive Vascular Diagnosis. Yearbook Medical pp 79-93.
13. Kupper CA, et al. Spectral Analysis of the Femoral Artery for Identification of Iliac Artery Lesions. Bruit 8: 157-63 June 1984
14. Flanigan DP et al. Utility of wide and narrow blood pressure cuffs in the hemodynamic assessment of aortoiliac disease. Surg 92: 16-20, 1982
15. Harris LM, Koerner NA, Curl GR, Ricotta JJ. Active pedal plantarflexion: a hemodynamic measurement of claudication. J Vasc Technol 19(3): 115-118,1995

CHAPTER 4: PHYSIOLOGIC CASE STUDIES

Several case studies are presented below for interpretation practice. The graphics in each exam have been enhanced to provide better "readability", increased font size, etc. Patient demographic information has been removed. Whenever possible, pertinent clinical information has been provided, as well as correlative information.

Try to make your own diagnosis prior to reading the explanation in "discussion" following each case study. There is a tendency to "over-read" physiologic studies, so remember the objective is to answer the following clinical questions:

1) Is the objective evidence for arterial occlusive disease?

2) Is the disease, if present, causing the patient's symptoms?

3) How severe is the disease?

4) What is the region of disease: aortoiliac, femoral -popliteal, or popliteal-tibial?

Some case studies will include both PVR and pressure data and CW-Doppler segmental waveforms and pressure data for comparison of the different methods. Acquiring both PVRs and Doppler waveforms is usually redundant and not necessary.

INTERPRETATION TIPS:

Step #1: look at ABIs first.

Step #2: confirm that ankle waveforms correlate with ankle pressures. If the pressures are abnormal, the waveforms should be abnormal as well).

Step #3: determine disease location (inflow versus infrainguinal), by assessing thigh PVR s (or CFA waveforms), and thigh pressures (if obtained).

Step #4: determine multi-level versus single level disease.

Step #5: determine disease severity, and if disease is related to the patient's condition.

Step #6: Remember the goals stated above, and don't try to "over-read" the studies.

NOTE: The term "biphasic" originally was used to describe the sound of a Doppler signal that lacked 3 component sounds (triphasic). Because there is considerable confusion regarding what constitutes a "biphasic" waveform, the term should be abandoned and not used to describe Doppler waveform morphology; use multiphasic, atypical or abnormal, and monophasic.

Study #1a. Full segmental PVR and pressure study.

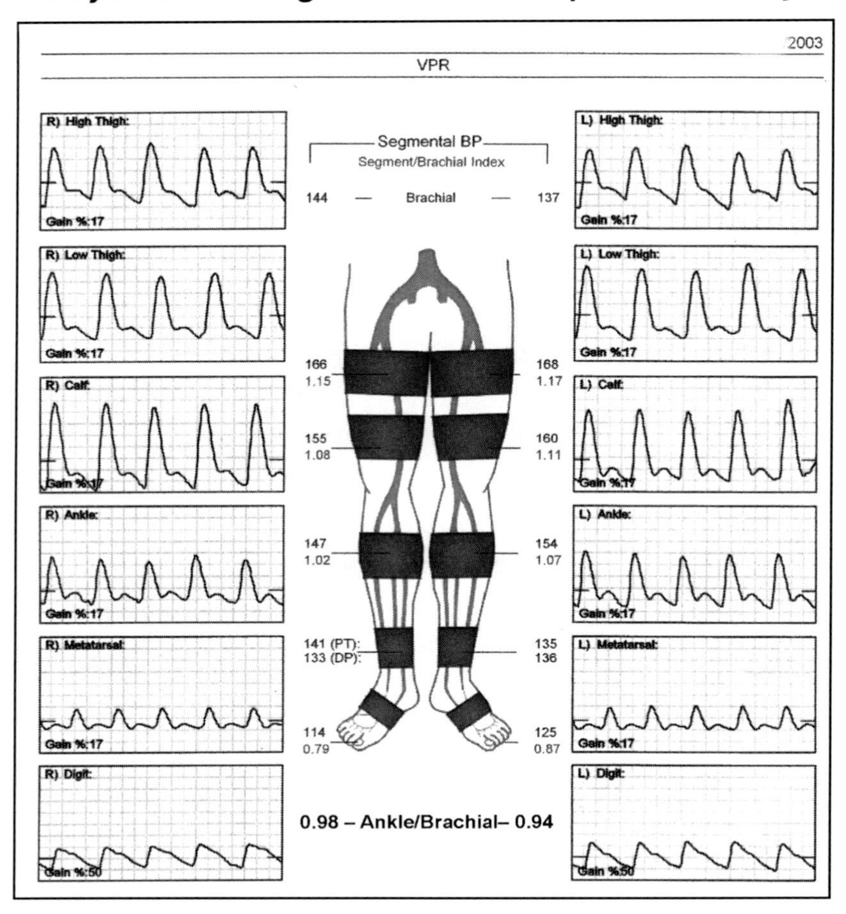

Study included PVRs from upper thigh, lower thigh, calf, ankle, metatarsal and great toe. Four-cuff segmental pressures and toe pressures were also obtained.

Study #1b. CW- Doppler exam from the same patient.

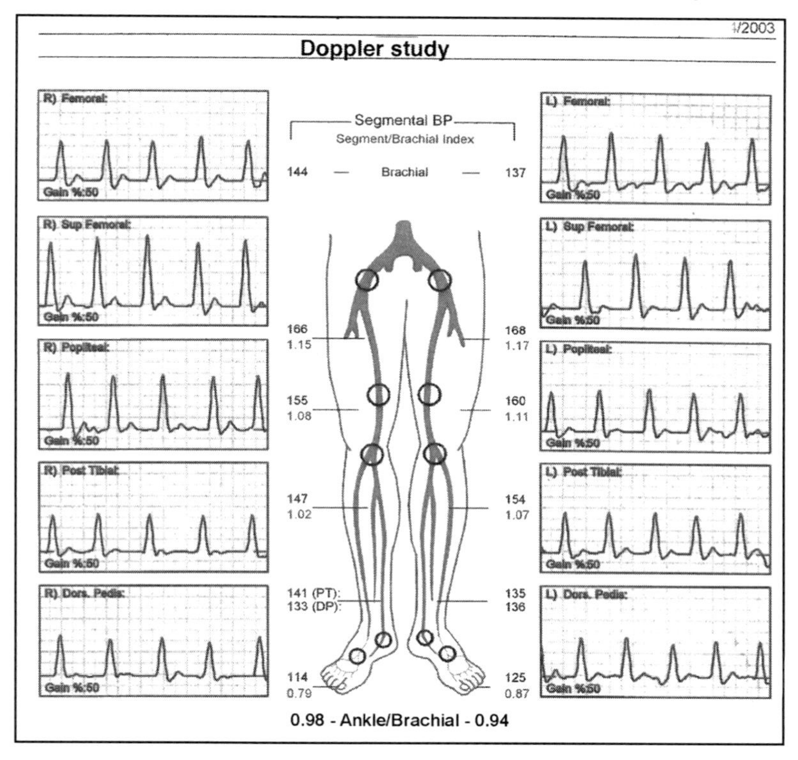

Study included CW-Doppler waveforms obtained from the CFA, SFA, Popliteal artery, PTA and DPA. Four-cuff segmental pressures and toe pressures were also obtained

Discussion: PVRs (VPRs) show pronounced reflective waves; ABIs and toe/brachial index (TBI) are normal. High-thigh pressures are normal and are higher than brachial pressures due to the "high-thigh cuff artifact". The metatarsal and great toe PVR amplitude is reduced, due to the gain or scale being too low for these sites. The Doppler study demonstrated normal waveforms at all sites. **Normal resting physiologic study, bilaterally.**

Study #2a.

Patient: D.S.

- 56-year-old male presents with progressive history of left buttock, thigh and calf claudication which presently limits walking to 2 blocks.
- Hx of smoking 1-2 ppd, recently quit.
- Hx of HT and angina. HX of coronary angioplasty.

PVR study with 4-cuff pressure assessment.

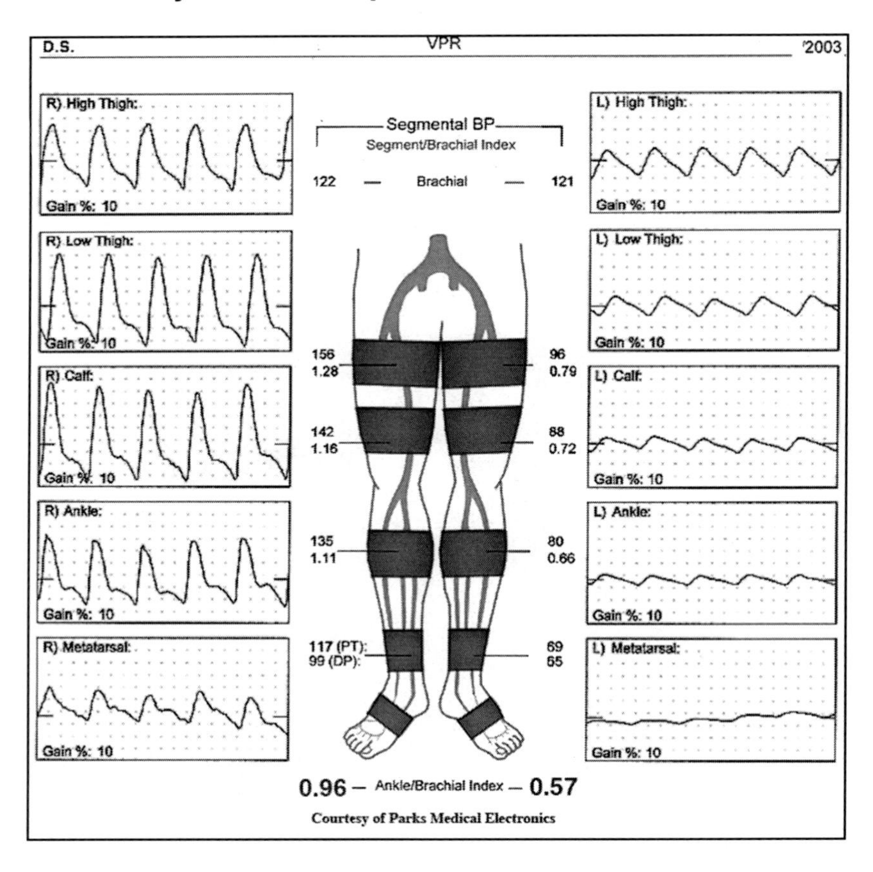

Courtesy of Parks Medical Electronics

Study #2b.
D.S., Same Patient

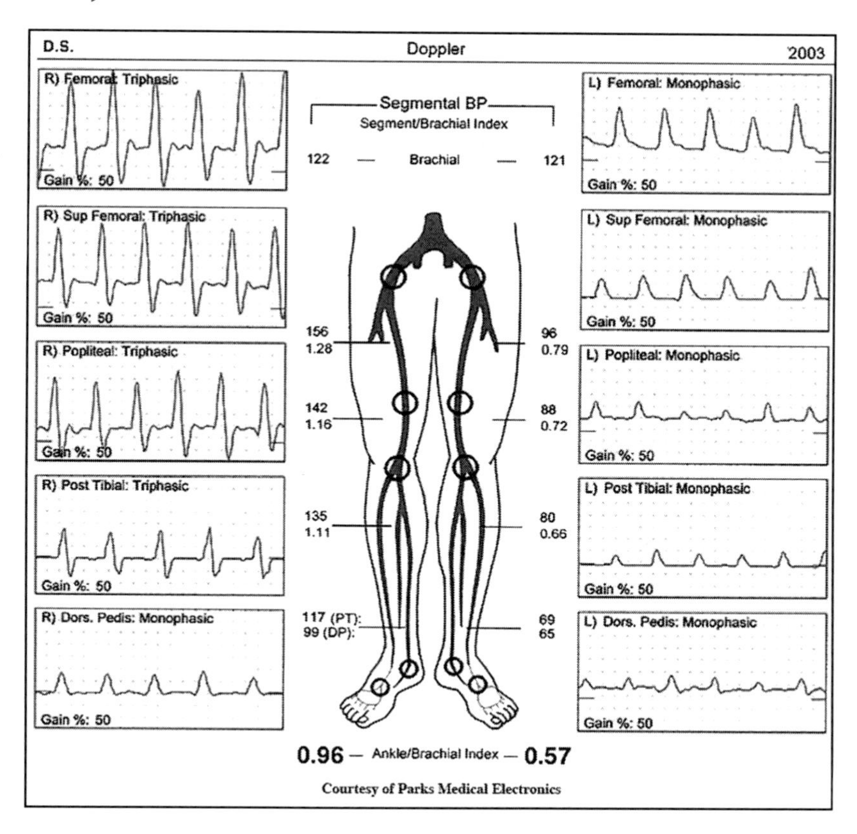

Courtesy of Parks Medical Electronics

Discussion: D.S. - Doppler and pressure portion of study

- The right ABI is 0.96 and normal; the left is 0.57 and abnormal.
- The left high-thigh pressure is decreased: this combined with the abnormal waveform suggests inflow (aorto-iliac) disease.
- Segmental pressures are normal on right (upper thigh with “high-thigh cuff artifact”).
- PVRs are normal on the right side demonstrating good amplitude and reflected waves at all sites.

- The left upper thigh PVR is abnormal with loss of amplitude (compared to the contralateral side) and no reflected wave. An abnormal PVR at the high-thigh level usually indicates inflow disease. PVR abnormality persists at all distal locations.
- In study 2b, Doppler waveforms are normal on the right side demonstrating triphasic pattern. However, the right dorsalis pedis waveform is somewhat abnormal and the pressure is reduced. This may indicate tibial disease in the anterior tibial or DPA, or it may be due to a small, atrophic DPA, a common finding.
- The left common femoral artery Doppler waveform is abnormal, and abnormal flow patterns persist at all distal sites. This would suggest inflow, or aorto-iliac disease on left.

Impression:

⇒ No evidence of arterial occlusive disease in right leg.

⇒ Right PVRs and Doppler waveforms are normal

⇒ Left ABI is abnormal. PVR and Doppler waveforms indicate moderate to severe aortoiliac disease in left leg.

Study #3.

Patient: W.W.

- This 82-year-old female presented with an ulcer on her left lateral ankle. Pulses: right CFA 2+, right Pop 2+, right DPA 1 +, right PTA 2 +; left CFA 2+, pulses below were absent.
- No history of smoking, MI or DM. History of hypertension.

Doppler and Segmental Pressure Study

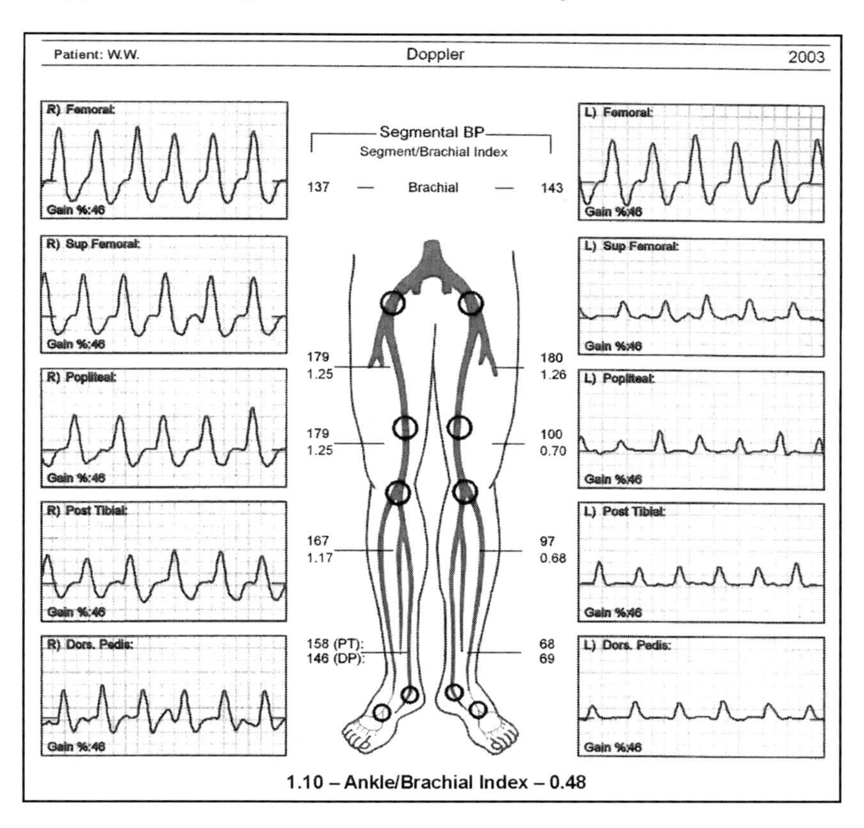

Discussion: Patient W.W.

- The right ABI (1.1) is normal. Doppler waveforms are multiphasic at all sites and are normal. The Doppler waveforms do not exhibit a pronounced third (triphasic) component in the diastolic portion of the cardiac cycle, but this often seen in otherwise normal patients. This may result from the Doppler probe angle being too high, or if wall compliance is poor.

- The left ABI is abnormal (0.48) and is in the range of multilevel disease or long segment occlusion. The left CFA Doppler wave is similar to right and is multiphasic. The SFA, POP and tibial waves are monophasic and abnormal.
- High-thigh pressures are normal bilaterally (both have the high-thigh cuff artifact). A significant pressure drop occurs between the left high-thigh and low-thigh cuff level.
- An additional pressure drop occurs at the ankle, but there is no degradation of the waveforms, so the significance is questionable.
- Patient was unable to perform stress exercise. Stress testing was also ill-advised in a patient with a potentially ischemic leg ulcer.

Impression:

⇒ No significant inflow disease.

⇒ Moderate to severe left femoro-popliteal disease, with a question of tibial involvement.

⇒ Resting study in right leg is normal.

Study #4.

Patient: B.M.

- A 90-year-old female presented with gangrenous toes in right foot.
- Pertinent medical history was unavailable.
- Pulses were absent in the right leg; left leg 1^+ at CFA, pulses were absent at other sites.

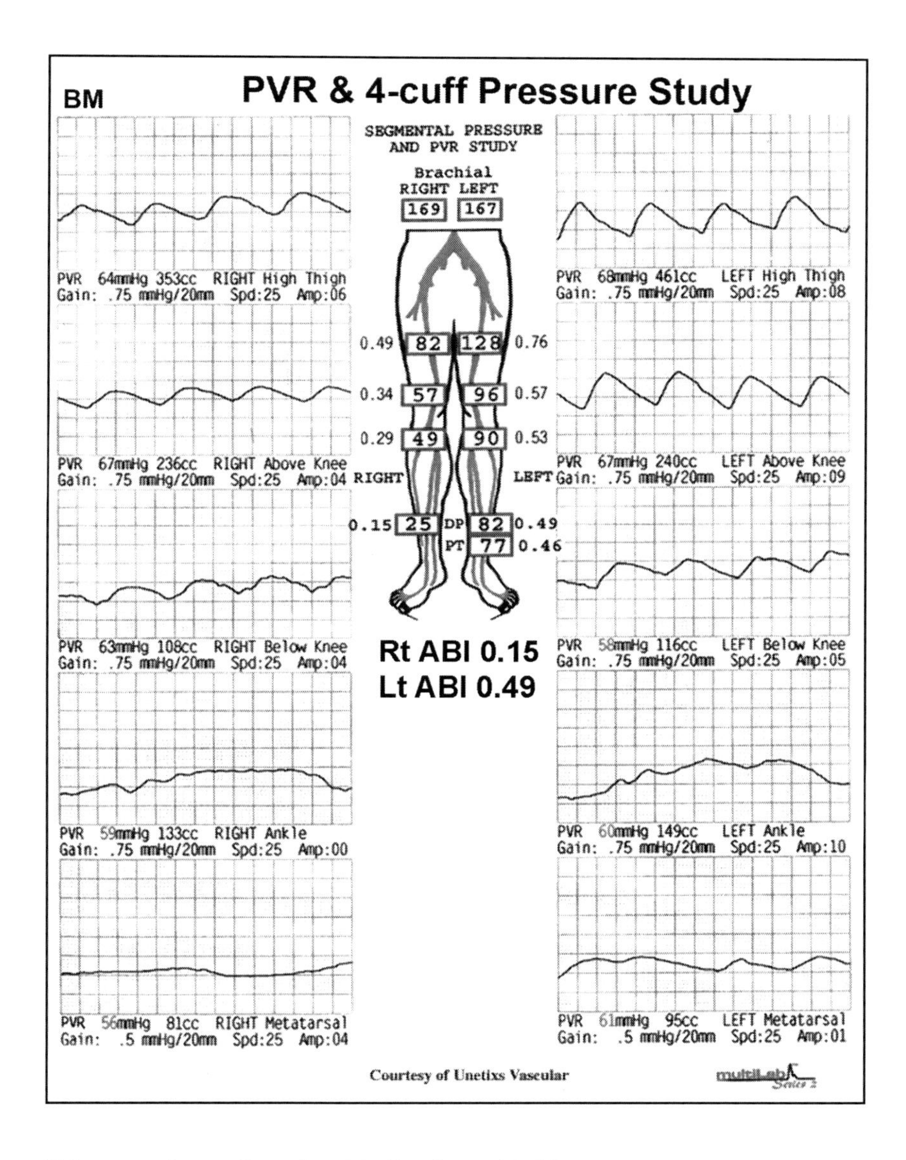

Discussion: Study #4. Patient B.M.

- ABIs are abnormal bilaterally (right 0.15, left 0.49), and in the ischemic range on the right.
- PVRs are abnormal at both upper thighs, indicating bilateral inflow disease, right > left.

- There is a decrease in PVR amplitude between the right calf and ankle. There is also a decrease in amplitude on the left side below the low-thigh level. This would suggest bilateral femoro-popliteal disease. However, PVRs are often unreliable for concomitant disease assessment distal to severe inflow disease.
- Segmental pressures are abnormal at the upper thigh bilaterally, right > left. This alone could be due to SFA disease or inflow disease (abnormal high-thigh pressure has only a 42% positive predictive value for iliac disease [5]) but it is consistent with abnormal inflow PVRs.
- Significant pressure decrease at the low-high on the right, and calf on the left is consistent with SFA or popliteal disease. A 25 mmHg pressure drop at the right ankle suggests tibial involvement as well.

Patient BM, Impression:

⇒ Right side: Severe ischemia right leg, severe aortoiliac disease, with probable femoro-popliteal disease. Cannot rule out tibial involvement.

⇒ Left side: moderate aortoiliac and femoro-popliteal disease.

Comment: The interpretation of pressures and waveforms on this study is complex, but remember the goals of physiologic testing. The questions answered include: the patient has arterial occlusive disease; it's severe and most likely causing her symptoms (gangrene), and it's multilevel disease.

Study #5.

Patient: B.S.

This 78-year-old female presented with recent onset right hip and leg pain soon after she started to walk. She was limited to walking 1 block. There was no history of MI, CVA, DM, HT, vascular surgeries or smoking.

She had been an active walker prior to the recent onset of discomfort.

- She has a known history of bilateral SFA stenoses diagnosed several years prior.
- The femoral artery disease was thought to be due to a form of arteritis related to polymyalgia rheumatica. She was treated with steroids and an active walking program. Her symptoms improved over the course of several months to a point that she was not limited by claudication.

PVR and 4-Cuff segmental pressure study

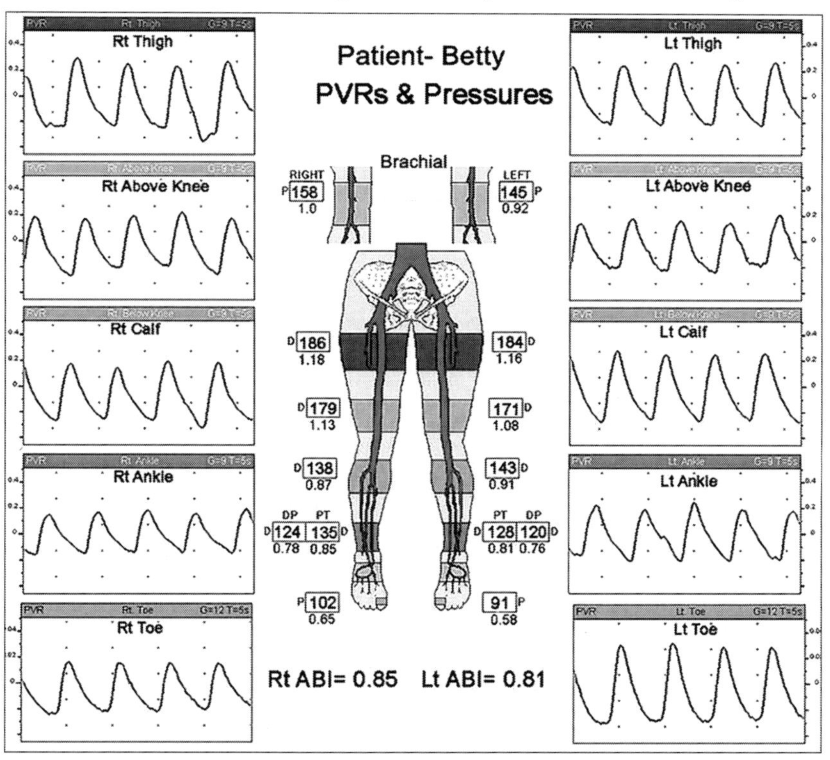

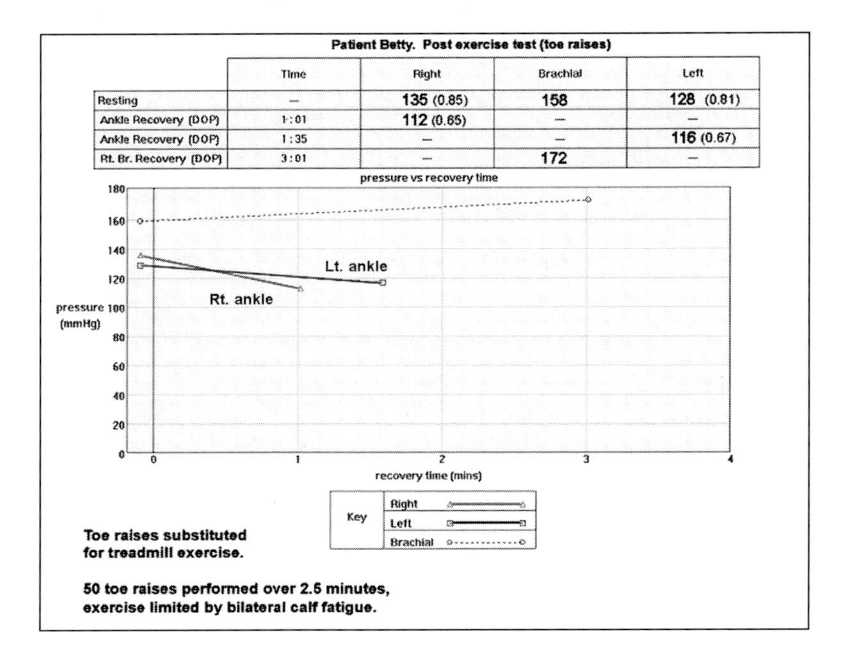

Patient Betty. Post exercise test (toe raises)

	Time	Right	Brachial	Left
Resting	–	135 (0.85)	158	128 (0.81)
Ankle Recovery (DOP)	1:01	112 (0.65)	–	–
Ankle Recovery (DOP)	1:35	–	–	116 (0.67)
Rt. Br. Recovery (DOP)	3:01	–	172	–

Toe raises substituted for treadmill exercise.

50 toe raises performed over 2.5 minutes, exercise limited by bilateral calf fatigue.

Discussion: Study #5. Patient B.S.

Resting study.

- Four-cuff pressure and PVR method used.
- ABIs are abnormal bilaterally (0.85 on right, 0.81 on left). The highest pressure value was used for the reported ABI.
- The high-thigh pressures are 30 mmHg above the brachial pressure (high-thigh cuff pressure artifact) and are normal. This rules out significant inflow disease.
- Although there appears to be a slight pressure drop between high-thigh and above knee cuffs, the drop between the above knee and calf cuffs is significant bilaterally.
- The pressure decrease at the ankles is within 20 mmHg of the calf pressures, so this is not significant.
- PVRs appear to be mildly abnormal at all sites.
- The resting study would suggest mild to moderate femoral–popliteal disease, bilaterally.

Exercise Stress test.

- The patient was unable to walk on the treadmill due to pain in right hip when standing. Toe raises were performed as a substitute for treadmill with a reasonably good effort.
- Ankle pressures immediately following the 2.5 minute exercise period were decreased bilaterally, with the right ankle at 112 mmHg and the left at 116 mmHg, down from 135 mmHg and 128 mmHg respectively. Serial pressures were not obtained.

Color duplex imaging demonstrated proximal SFA stenoses of both legs. Noted were atypically large profunda femoral arteries, often seen when good collateralization has occurred in the presence of SFA obstruction. This may account for the nearly normal PVRs in both legs.

Summary: Although this patient has arterial occlusive disease, it is unlikely that this is the source of her symptoms. Her post-exercise ankle pressures did not reflect an ischemic condition necessary to explain a vascular etiology for claudication. Her ABIs had, in fact, improved since her studies from several years before.

Computerized tomography revealed a narrow spinal canal at the L-5 level.

This case demonstrates the importance of physiologic testing in assessing the ***effect*** of disease on overall limb perfusion.

Study #6.

Patient: J.D.

- This 76-year-old male presented with 1 year history of right ankle, knee and hip pain when walking, relieved by rest. History of osteoarthritis in feet.
- History of hypertension, hyperlipidemia, MI, and smoking (quit 5 years ago).

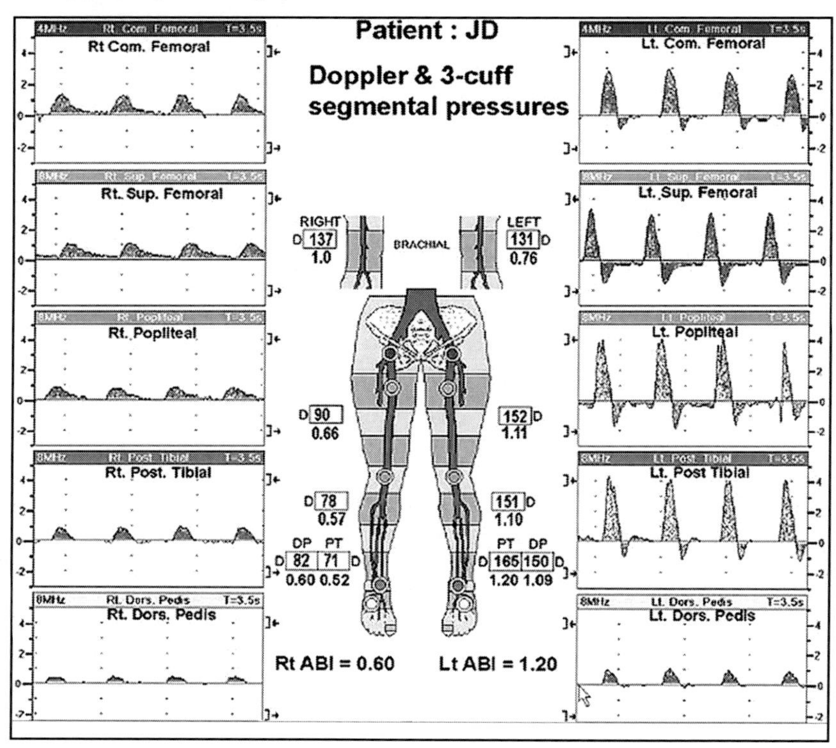

Discussion: Study #6. Patient J.D.

- Three-cuff pressure test with segmental Doppler spectral analysis.
- Right ABI is abnormal (0.60), ABI on left is normal.
- Abnormal, monophasic CW Doppler waveform at the right CFA suggests significant inflow disease.
- Doppler waveforms are persistently abnormal distally in the right leg.

- Right thigh pressure is low (90mmHg) without additional significant drop to calf.
- Left side Doppler waveforms and pressures are normal. However, the left DPA waveform is diminished, probably due to a small vessel with lower flow.

Impression: significant aortoiliac disease on right; normal study on left leg.

Study #7.

Patient: McG ----No history available.

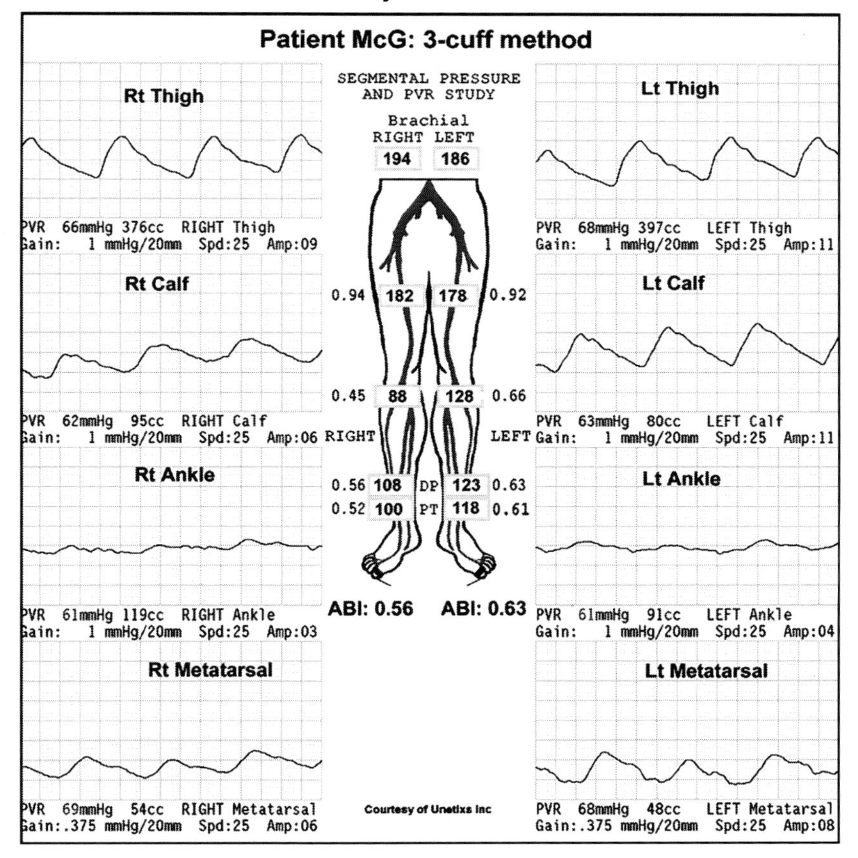

Discussion: Study #7.

- The ABIs are abnormal bilaterally.
- Thigh pressures are normal for the 3-cuff pressure method

- .A significant pressure drop occurred at both calves.
- PVRs at both thighs are marginally normal (but, there are no distinct reflective waves).
- PVR waveforms are abnormal at the calf level bilaterally, right greater than left. (Typically in a three-cuff method using a 17 cm thigh cuff, the calf PVR amplitude is higher than the thigh PVR in normal perfusion).
- Metatarsal PVRs are higher in amplitude compared to the ankle PVRs; probably due to a difference in PVR gain (scale).

Note: There are a few technical problems in this study.

1)The ankle PVRs and the pressures do not agree. The PVRs are almost flatline and the pressures are over 100 mmHg. One would expect a lower pressure at the ankle level with nearly flat-line PVRs.

2) The right calf pressure was measured at 88 mmHg and pressure increased at the ankle to 108 mmHg. Pressures may decrease in the presence of disease, but they don't increase (the exception being a case where pressures are artificially elevated due to calcified tibial arteries). The technologist should have repeated the pressures and PVRs at the ankle level.

Study #8.

Patient: R.S.

- A 53-year-old male presented with history of stable, bilateral intermittent hip, buttock and thigh claudication limiting walking to 3 blocks.
- Hx of angina, HT, and smoking 1-2 ppd.
- Hx of coronary artery bypass graft (CABG).
- Pulses CFA 1^+, POP 0, PTA 1^+, DPA 1^+, bilaterally.

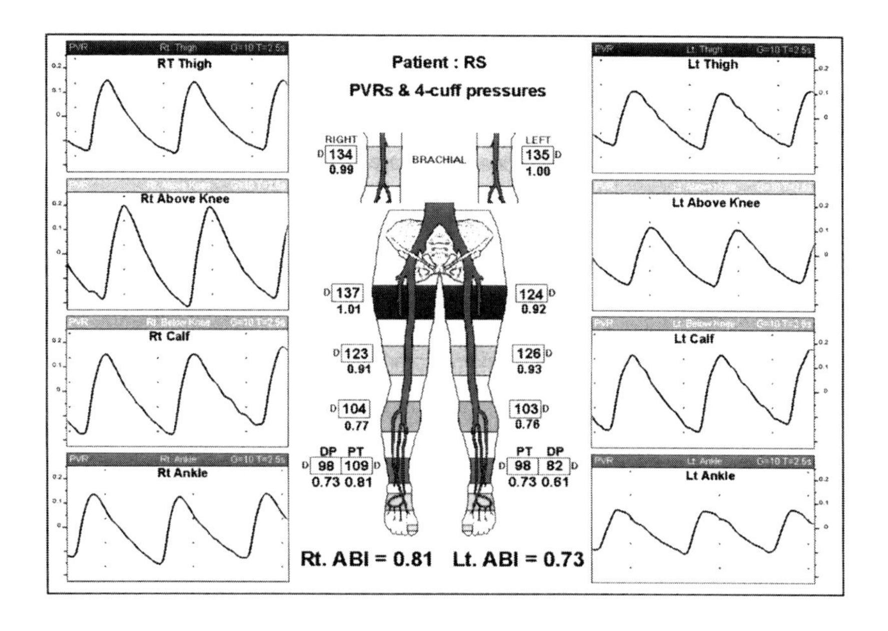

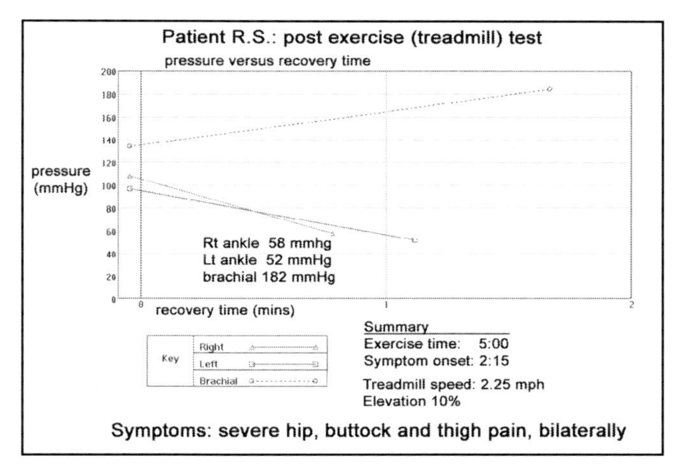

Discussion: RS Study

- ABIs are abnormal bilaterally.
- Upper thigh pressures are abnormal (they should be 20- 30 mmHg above brachial pressure).

- PVRs are borderline abnormal on the right upper thigh, with mildly abnormal waveform on the left upper thigh.
- Distal PVRs are mildly abnormal and similar to thigh waveforms.
- There is a borderline significant pressure drop at the calf level bilaterally; this may suggest femoro-popliteal disease, but there is no significant change in PVR morphology.

Post exercise:

- Patient walked for 5 minutes but experienced severe hip, buttock and thigh pain bilaterally.
- Ankle pressures dropped to 58 mmHg (ABI 0.32), and 52 mmHg (ABI 0.29) in right and left ankles respectively.
- Post exercise ankle pressures less than 60 mmHg suggest a vascular cause for the claudication.
- **Impression:** Moderate aortoiliac disease bilaterally resulting in vascular claudication. Question of mild femoro-popliteal disease bilaterally.

Color Duplex Imaging revealed bilaterally severe common iliac artery stenoses.

Study #9.

Patient: J.F.

- A 34-year-old male presented with acute onset right calf claudication.
- No symptoms in left leg.
- Hx of Aorta to right common femoral bypass one year before.
- Pulses at Rt. CFA, POP, DPA, PTA were absent. Left leg pulses were 2^+ at all sites

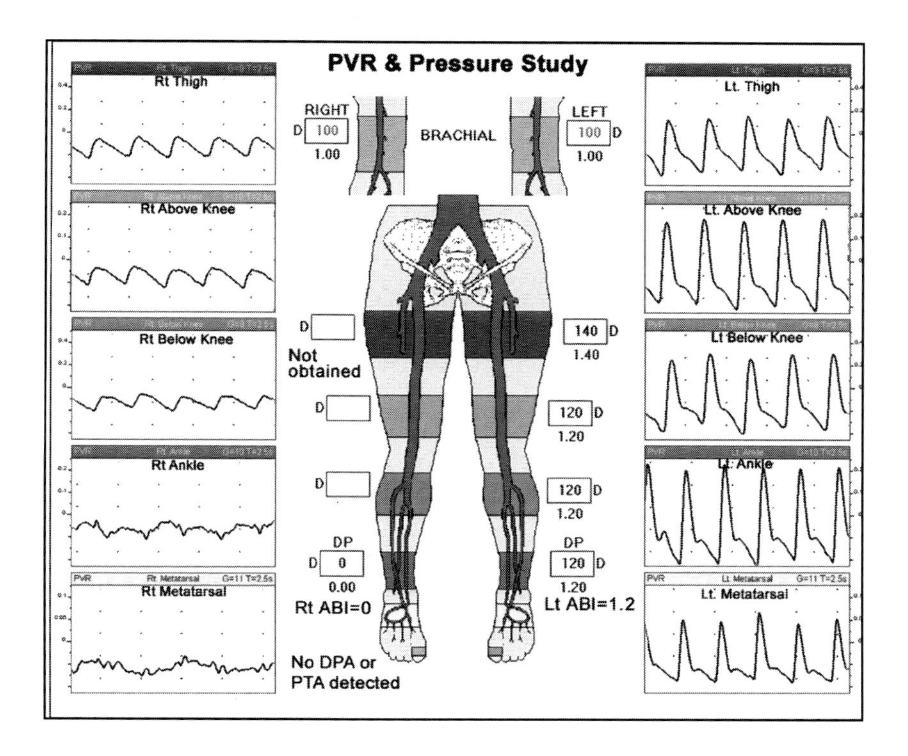

Discussion: Study #9 Patient J.F.

- Normal PVRs and ABI on left side.
- Unable to obtain pressures in right leg (no flow detectable by Doppler in either pedal arteries).
- Abnormal PVR at right upper thigh indicates severe inflow disease.
- The fact that he has a graft on the right side suggests graft occlusion.
- Angiography revealed a thrombosed aorto-femoral graft. Patient underwent a successful thrombectomy.

Study #10.

Patient: Danny

This study was obtained on a volunteer during a teaching exercise.

Patient was a 54 year-old male with a history of type 2 diabetes.

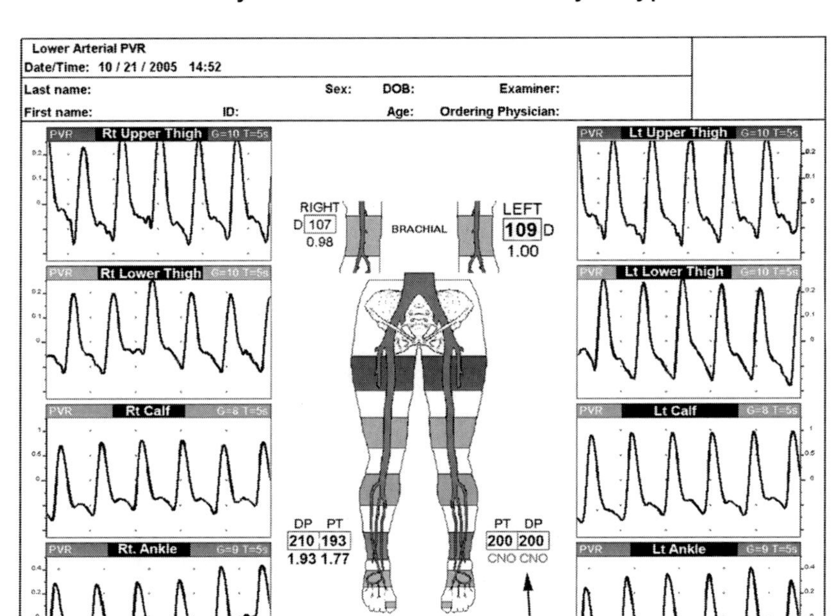

Discussion: Study #10. Patient: Danny.

- The ABI on the right is very high (1.93). The left ABI was unobtainable, as the pedal vessels could not be compressed or occluded during pressure acquisition. Although 200 mmHg is entered as the left ankle pressure, the CNO designation, for "Cannot Occlude" (a modality of this particular PVR system) indicates that cuff pressure exceeded that amount, and the Doppler signal was not obliterated. Note that the brachial pressure is only 109 mmHg.
- The high ankle pressures on the right and the inability to occlude on the left indicates the presence of calcified tibial vessels, or calcific medial sclerosis.
- The PVRs are normal at all sites and the toe/brachial index (TBI) is normal bilaterally.
- Other than calcified tibial arteries, this is a normal study.

Study #11- Example of a technically flawed study.

This is a limited, physiologic study (option 1) to include ABIs and PVRs from the ankle level. Review this study and try to identify the error(s) before reading the discussion below.

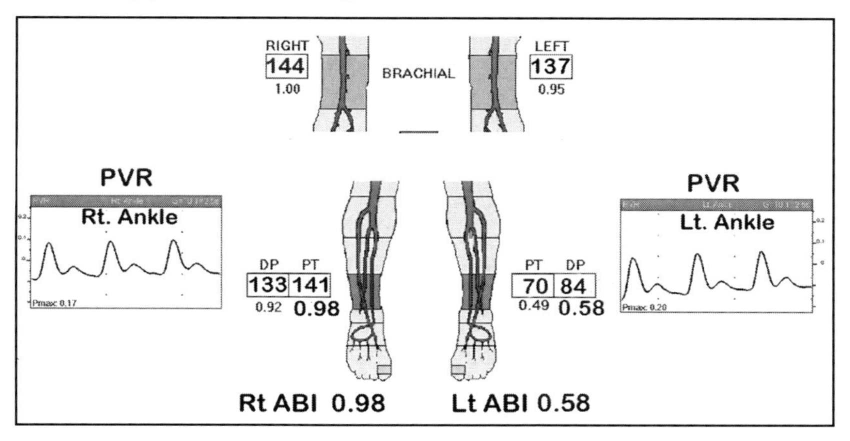

The ankle/brachial index on the right is normal and the ankle pressures (PTA and DPA) are within 15% of each other. The pulse volume recording is of good quality and exhibits a normal profile with a prominent reflective wave. The resting study on the right is unequivocally normal.

On the left, both ankle pressures and ABI (0.58) are abnormal; this would suggest moderate PAD in the left leg. However, the PVR is normal and similar to the right ankle PVR. The data is inconsistent, and the study is flawed on the left leg with a probable technical error in ankle pressure acquisition.

At the ankle level, pressures and PVR data should match, i.e., if ankle pressures are abnormal the PVR (and/or Doppler waveform) should also be abnormal. Conversely, if the ankle pressures are normal, we'd expect the PVRs to be normal. As discussed in earlier chapters, errors can and do occur in obtaining limb pressures. It's very important that the technologist recognize when an error has occurred at the time of the exam. PVRs are less prone to technical error and it's very unlikely that a perfusion deficiency at the ankle will result in a normal PVR. In this (probably normal) study, the left ankle pressures should have been repeated.

A "check and balance" occurs when 2 pressures at each ankle are obtained (they should be similar), and by the addition of a PVR or Doppler waveform (should concur with the pressure data).

Study #12.

Patient: H.K.

This 59-year-old female presented with a progressive history of bilateral leg claudication that limited walking to 1-2 blocks. She has a history of a repaired dissecting thoracic aorta, and hypertension. No HX of MI, DM.

This is an older study from the days of PVR strip chart recording and cut-and-paste reports. Segmental PVRs and ABIs were obtained, and a post-exercise study was performed.

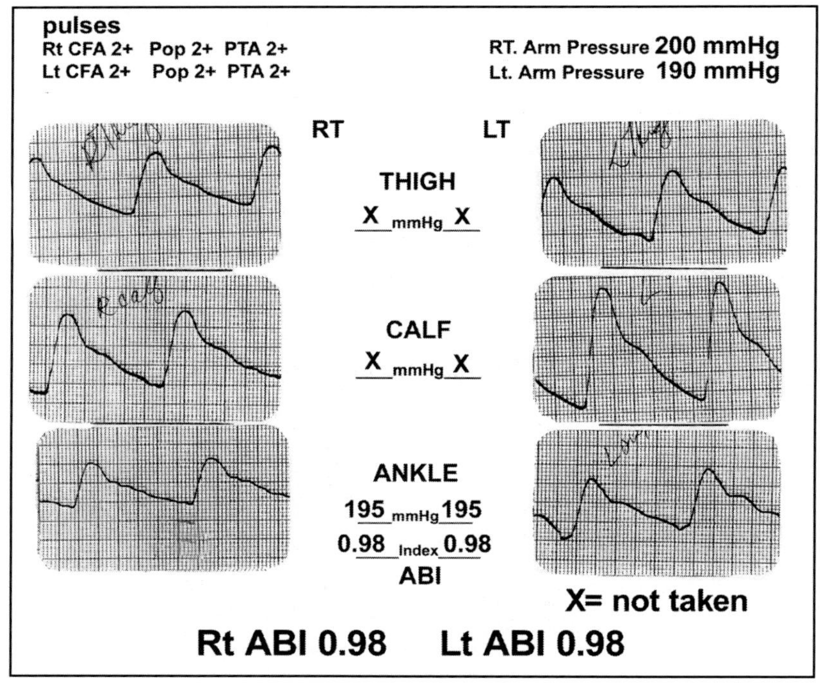

Resting ABIs are normal bilaterally, and PVRs are normal at all levels. Calf and ankle pressures were not obtained as the ankle pressures were normal. Despite a normal resting exam, the patient was exercised on a treadmill due to her complaint of claudication.

Treadmill speed was 1.5 MPH with a 10% grade. Bilateral leg fatigue limited walking to 1 min. 25 seconds.

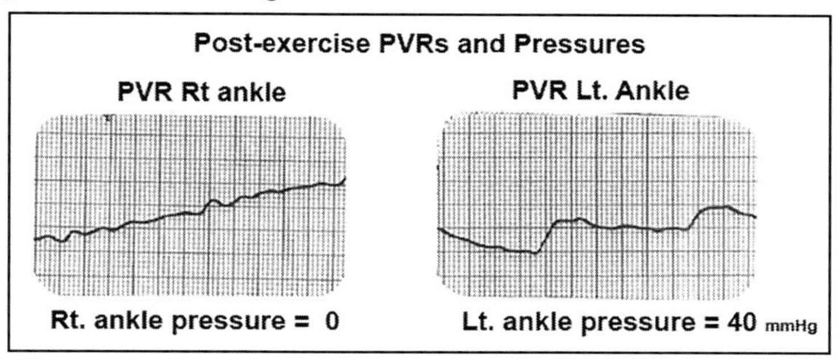

Post-exercise Rt. ankle pressure could not be obtained, as there was no detectable flow. A unilateral PVR was obtained to confirm the findings (it was flat-line). The left ankle pressure was 40 mmHg and had probably risen during the time it took to assess the right ankle. An abnormal PVR of the left ankle confirmed the finding of a low ankle pressure.

Discussion: Study #12. H.K.

This study demonstrates the important of treadmill exercise, particularly in patients that complain of claudication. The resting study was normal, but the patient had significant disease that become "hemodynamically" significant during exercise. According to the tenet of Poiseuille's law, a flow volume increase over a stenosis increases the pressure gradient, in this case, dramatically. Color duplex imaging revealed an abdominal aortic dissection with significant reduction in aortic lumen diameter. Proximal lesions have more impact on limb perfusion than distal obstruction, as there is no "opportunity" for collateral pathways.

Study #13. Patient: L.V.

68-year-old male referred for rest pain in left foot, and non-healing ulcer on left ankle. No other history available. ABIs and PVRs (3-cuff method with large 18 cm thigh cuff) were obtained.

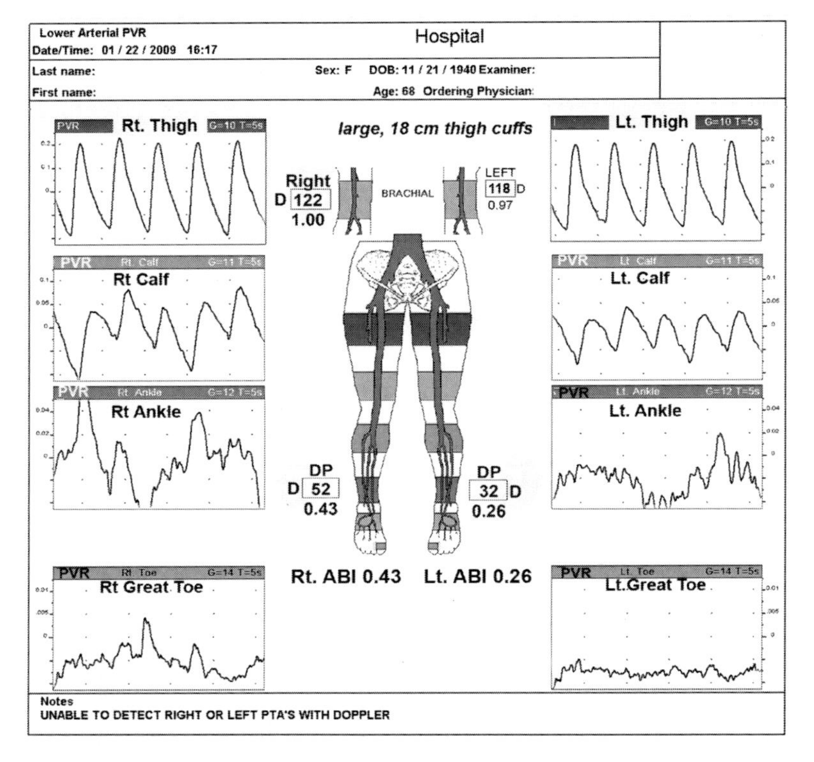

PVRs were non-diagnostic at ankle level so Doppler waveforms were obtained from the DPAs. No detectable flow in the PTAs.

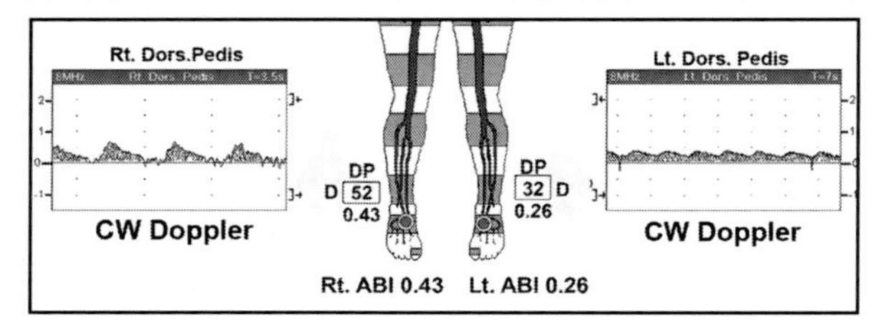

Inflow appears OK, but severe femoro-popliteal disease bilaterally, left greater than right. Left ulcer is unlikely to heal with ankle pressure less than 50 mmHg. Doppler waveforms in this case were superior to ankle PVRs. PVR inflation pressure (65 mmHg) may have obliterated flow in the ankles.

CHAPTER 5: ABBREVIATED, EFFICIENT, LOWER ARTERIAL PROTOCOLS

Noninvasive physiologic testing for arterial occlusive disease was developed prior to color duplex imaging, magnetic resonance angiography (MRA) and computerized tomography angiography (CTA). Before physiologic testing, the diagnosis of PAD was based on the history and physical exam and the painful contrast biplane angiography. Physiologic testing tried to provide the clinician with as much information as possible, consequently the test modalities were extensive, somewhat redundant and time consuming.

CTA and MRA are too expensive, and color duplex imaging is too time-consuming to be used as a screening test for PAD, but are important tools when used in conjunction with physiologic testing. They can provide information not obtainable with indirect pressures and waveforms, e.g., the exact site and extent of disease, and whether arteries are stenosed or occluded.

The following is a recommendation by this author for an efficient, cost-effective protocol which answers the important clinical questions. Two variations will be discussed; one is based on pulse volume recording, the other on Doppler waveform analysis. *Only one of these protocol variations needs to be followed.*

Keep in mind the goals of testing:

1. Is there evidence for PAD?
2. If present, is it mild, moderate or severe?
3. What is the region of disease? Is it aortoiliac, femoro-popliteal, popliteal-tibial, or multiple segments?
4. If disease is present, is it responsible for the patient's symptoms?

Goals #1 & 2 of physiologic testing.

Answer this clinical question: *Is there objective evidence for peripheral arterial disease? And if present, how severe?*

I. PVR-BASED PROTOCOL

Perform limited, bilateral noninvasive physiologic studies of the lower extremities (CPT code 93922).

- Using a CW Doppler and pressure system, obtain systolic pressures from both arms and ankles, in the following sequence. Rt. arm, Rt. PTA, Rt. DPA, Lt. PTA, Lt. DPA, Lt. arm, right arm.
  - ⇒ If the difference between the 2 right arm measurements exceeds 10 mmHg, the first measurement should be disregarded and only the second measurement used.
  - ⇒ If there is more than a 15-20 mmHg difference between the PTA and DPA pressures on same ankle, repeat the ankle pressures.
  - ⇒ If the ankle pressures cannot be obtained due to calcified vessels, obtain great toe pressures and calculate the TBI.
- Acquire pulse volume recordings (PVRs) from the ankles bilaterally. If these are non-diagnostic due to motion artifact, acquire CW Doppler waveforms from the 4 pedal arteries.
- If you prefer Doppler waveforms over PVR, acquire ankle Doppler waveforms instead of PVRs.
- Perform exercise stress test in appropriate (claudicating) patients, or in borderline normal patients.
- *Don't* exercise patients with rest pain, ankle ulceration, ABIs less than 0.4, or with other contraindications (see chapter 3).

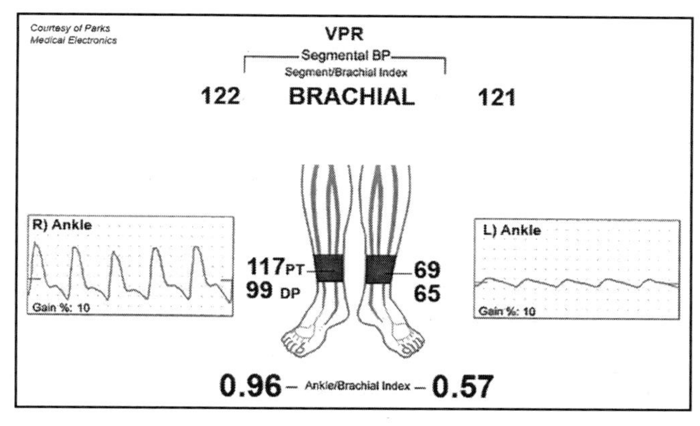

The study above is a limited, bilateral physiologic study with PVR (VPR) demonstrating moderate PAD in the left leg; the right leg is normal (at rest).

The patient (above) has moderate PAD in the left leg, the right leg is normal (at rest). This information has been provided in a 15 minute examination. Questions #1 & 2 have been answered; the patient has moderate PAD in the left leg. Exercise stress testing at this point would confirm that PAD is causing claudication, although it is very likely, considering the resting ankle pressures.

The terms mild, moderate, severe are subjective, but can be loosely applied based on resting ABIs. "Mild" would indicate a minimum decrease in ABI at rest and during exercise. ABIs of $\leq$ 0.3 would be indicative of "severe" disease. ABIs of 0.4 - 0.8 would be considered "moderate" disease.

Questions NOT answered in this abbreviated exam:

- What is the disease level - inflow or infrainguinal? (Is this important? If not, there is no need for a complete bilateral study).
- Is the disease single level or multilevel? (Is this important?)
- Is the disease causing the claudication? (Probably).

Goal #3: To determine the disease level, extend exam to a "complete, bilateral physiologic study."

- Add blood pressure cuffs to the calf and thigh, bilaterally. *(I'd recommend wrapping all cuffs, ankle through thigh, at the beginning of the exam. There is diagnostic and financial benefit to performing a complete bilateral study).*
- Obtain pulse volume recordings at 3 or more levels. Ankle PVRs have already been acquired, so obtain thigh (1 or 2 cuffs) and calf PVRs (add metatarsal and toe PVRs, if warranted).
- As of this writing, segmental pressures from 3 or more locations are not required if PVRs are performed as part of the "complete study" CPT 93923.

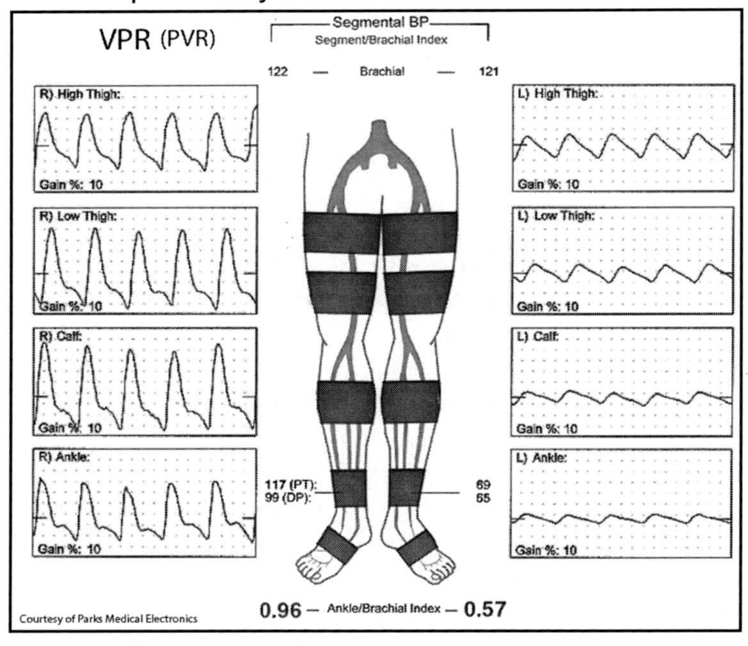

The study above is a complete, bilateral physiologic study. It's similar to the previous, limited study demonstration, but PVRs have been added at the calf, low thigh and high thigh. Abnormal left upper thigh VPR indicates that this patient has left inflow disease (left iliac disease). Right side is normal.

Question #3 has been answered; The disease level appears to be left inflow disease. *This information was provided with an additional 5-10 minutes of exam time. Total exam time to this point is approximately 20-30 minutes.*

<u>Would segmental pressures help in this case to define disease level?</u>

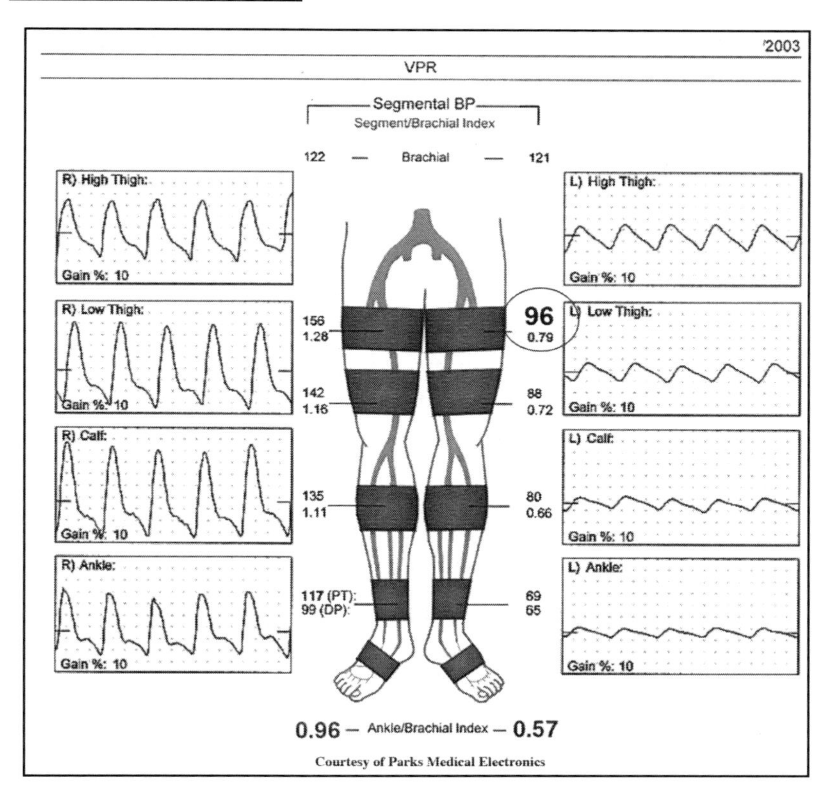

Courtesy of Parks Medical Electronics

Full segmental pressures were added to the PVR/ABI study. The high pressure in the right thigh is normal and demonstrates a cuff artifact. Left thigh pressure is 26 mmHg lower than the arm, and is abnormal.

Did thigh pressures help here, NO! Thigh pressures are painful for many patients, and because there is confusion about high-thigh pressure interpretation (some patients have the "high-thigh cuff artifact", while others don't), the best method to assess inflow is with thigh PVRs or common femoral artery

Doppler waveforms.

⇒ A low thigh pressure can be due to femoral disease or aortoiliac disease.

⇒ The additional time and effort of segmental pressures has not provided any additional, useful information in this case.

Questions NOT answered in this exam at this point:

- Is the vascular inflow disease causing the patient's claudication?
- How do we answer this clinical question?
  1. Assumption (low resting ankle pressure on left).
  2. Perform exercise stress test.

Treadmill Stress Test

- Determine if the patient is a candidate for treadmill exercise. Carefully screen for contraindications and follow the guidelines discussed in Chapter 3.
- Record treadmill speed, elevation, symptoms and time of onset, maximal walking time, and time to recover.
- Move the patient to the exam bed ASAP after exercise.
- Some labs will leave the ankle (2) and arm (1) pressure cuffs on during exercise so that they do not have to be reapplied. Tape the cuffs so they don't flap around when the patient is walking.

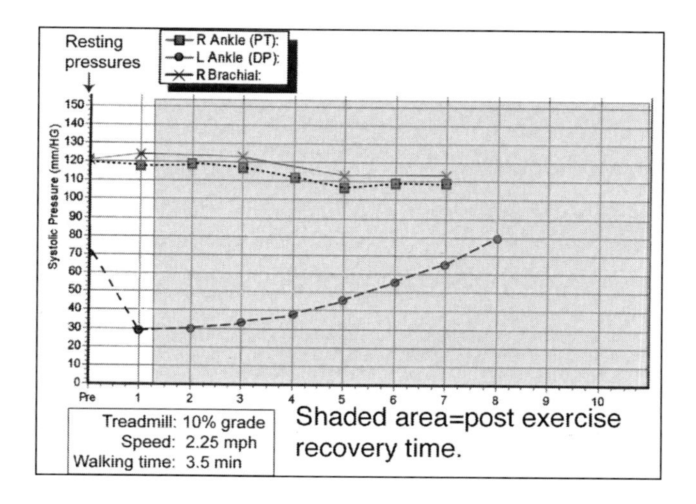

The post-exercise chart above demonstrates a significant pressure drop in the left ankle following exercise. Recovery time is 8 minutes.

Post treadmill exercise procedure.

⇒ Measure post-exercise ankle pressures, start with the symptomatic leg.

⇒ If ankle pressure is below 60 mmHg, it's a vascular cause for claudication.

⇒ If ankle pressures decrease, record ABIs at timed intervals until ankle pressures reach resting levels.

⇒ There is no need for serial pressure measurements if the initial post exercise ankle pressures are normal.

If the patient cannot tolerate the stress of the treadmill, perform toe raise test and measure ankle pressures after exercise. This method is more thoroughly demonstrated in Chapter 3.

If treadmill stress test is performed following the resting physiologic exam, the CPT code is 93924

II. DOPPLER WAVEFORM-BASED PROTOCOL

Some diagnostic labs use CW Doppler waveform analysis instead of PVRs. There are advantages and disadvantages for each modality, but the biggest disadvantage of Doppler waveforms is the high skill requirement. With poor technique, waveforms can be made to appear abnormal on an otherwise normal individual. Also, the transducer might be over the wrong artery. If you elect to use this "option" in any of the physiologic test protocols, you should carefully review the Doppler method section in the Instrumentation chapter.

This protocol is less "efficient" than PVR protocols, as it requires pressure acquisition from multiple limb sites, and Doppler waveforms, which are more difficult to acquire than PVRs.

Use the same logical steps as described earlier to answer the important clinical questions.

Perform limited, bilateral noninvasive physiologic studies of the lower extremities (CPT code 93922).

- Obtain ABIs in the following sequence: Rt. arm, Rt. PTA, Rt. DPA, Lt. PTA, Lt. DPA, Lt. arm, right arm.
  - ⇒ If the difference between the 2 right arm measurements exceeds 10 mmHg, the first measurement should be disregarded and only the second measurement used.
  - ⇒ If there is more than a 15-20 mmHg difference between the PTA and DPA pressures on same ankle, repeat the ankle pressures.
  - ⇒ If the ankle pressures cannot be obtained due to calcified vessels, obtain great toe pressures and calculate the TBI.

- Acquire and record CW Doppler waveforms from the PTA & DPA of each foot.

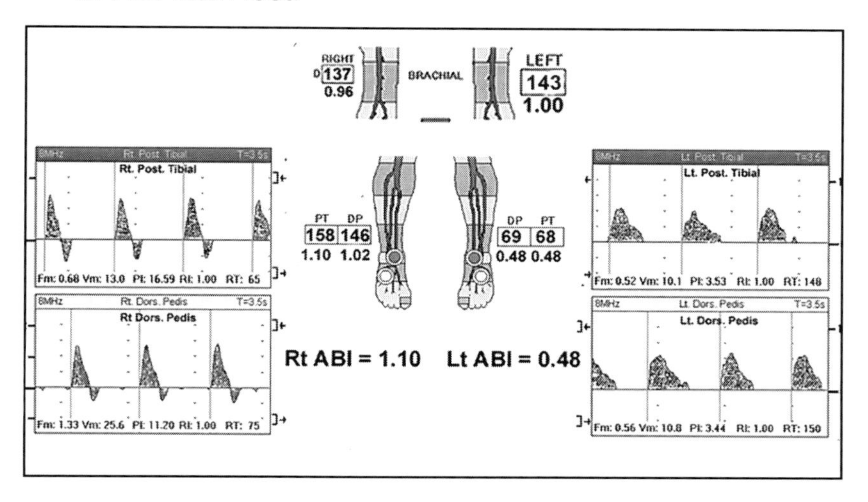

This is a limited physiologic study with the Doppler option for waveforms. On the left, the ABI and the pedal artery waveforms are abnormal. The right size is normal.

This study demonstrates PAD in the left leg, but with only information from the ankle, the location of disease is unknown.

To determine the region of disease, extend the exam to a complete physiologic study. *This will include Doppler waveforms* ***and*** *segmental pressures from 3 or more locations.* This is the definition of CPT code 93923.

Segmental Pressures

- Apply blood pressure cuffs to the calf, low thigh and high thigh bilaterally, as previously described. Wrap the cuffs as snugly as possible.
  - ⇒ If cuffs are loose, a large volume of air must go into the cuff during inflation to occlude the arteries. Inflation time can be very long, patient discomfort increases, and technical errors are more likely to occur.

- Position the Doppler over the PTA, or if the signal is weak, over the DPA.
- Inflate the calf cuff and record systolic pressure. Without moving the Doppler probe from the PTA or DPA, inflate the thigh cuffs and obtain systolic pressures.
- Obtain segmental pressures from the left leg in a similar fashion.
- If the ankle, and calf pressures are normal, logically, there is no need to obtain thigh pressures.

> Before you obtain thigh pressures on patients, I'd recommend that you have a colleague/coworker obtain a high and low thigh pressure on you. Some people can tolerate the "discomfort" well, for others it is extremely painful. If your supervising physician insist that you obtain thigh pressures (unnecessarily) on patients, ask that he or she volunteer for the test. It's important to understand what the patient is experiencing.

- Obtain toe pressures, if appropriate (history of diabetes, question of small vessel disease, or calcified tibial arteries). Toe pressures are not easily obtained in some patients due to poor toe cuff fit, or PPG sensor placement. Some labs perform toe pressures routinely if patients have a history of diabetes.
- Remove blood pressure cuffs.

Segmental Doppler Waveforms

- Waveforms from the PTA and DPA should already have been acquired.
- Obtain Doppler waveforms from the following sites:
  - ⇒ popliteal artery (behind the knee)
  - ⇒ superficial femoral artery (SFA) (mid thigh)

⇒ common femoral artery (CFA) at the groin crease.

The site sequence is not important, use whatever the system software dictates. Repeat on the contralateral side.

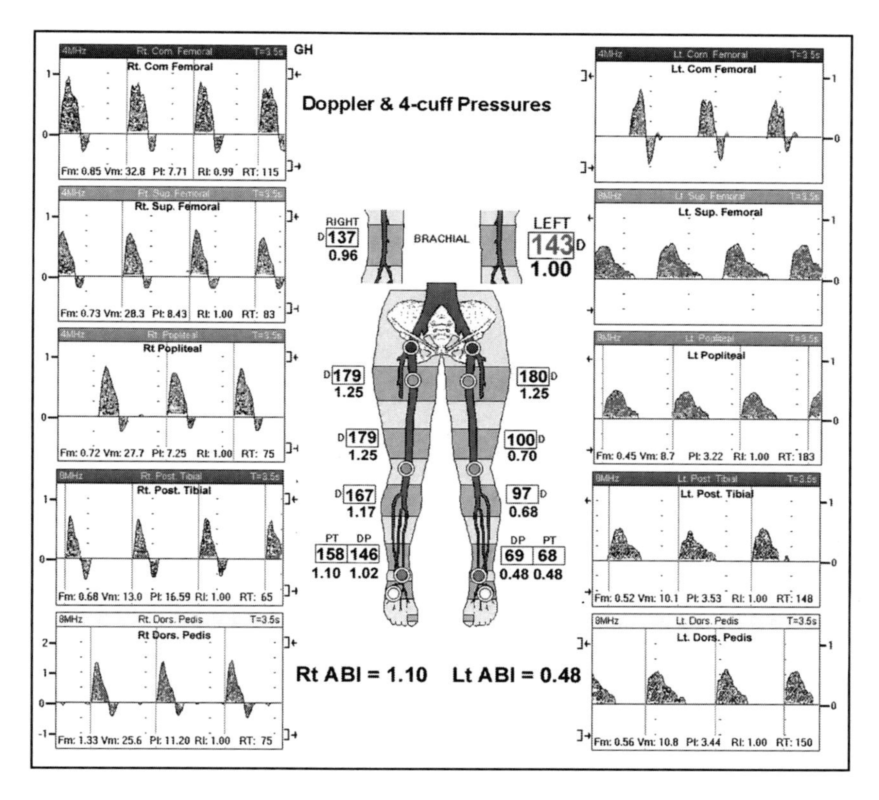

The study above is a complete, bilateral noninvasive physiologic study with segmental pressures and Doppler waveforms at 3 or more levels. This is an extension of the previous limited study. The CFA waveforms and high-thigh pressures are normal. There is a significant pressure drop at the left low thigh, and the SFA waveform is abnormal. The region of disease is the femoro-popliteal segment.

Treadmill Stress Test

- Determine if the patient is a candidate for treadmill exercise. Carefully screen for contraindications and follow the guidelines discussed in chapter 3.

- Record treadmill speed, elevation, symptoms and time of onset, maximal walking time, and time to recover.
- Move the patient to the exam bed ASAP after exercise.
- Some labs will leave the ankle (2) and arm (1) pressure cuffs on during exercise so that they do not have to be reapplied. Tape the cuffs to they don't flap around.
- Starting with the symptomatic leg, record bilateral ankle pressures. Record arm pressure from one arm. Measure ABIs serially until the lowest ankle pressure has returned to baseline, pre-exercise levels.

CHAPTER 6: ARTERIAL PHYSIOLOGIC TESTING: UPPER EXTREMITIES

UPPER ARTERIAL ANATOMY

1. Brachiocephalic a. (innominate) - right side only.
2. Subclavian a.
   - Left: originates at the aortic arch.
   - Right: originates at the brachiocephalic artery.

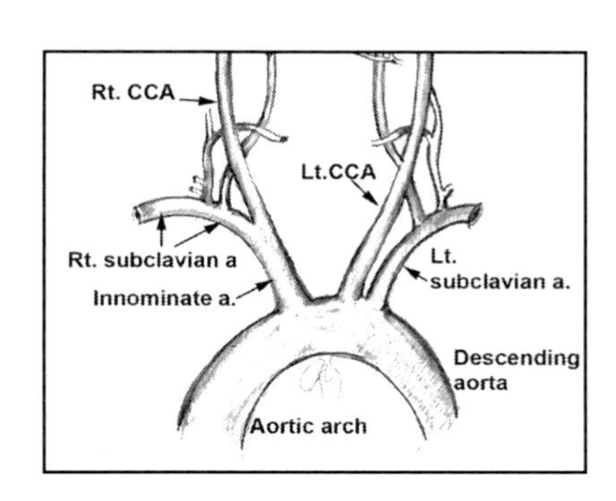

3. Axillary a.- from the first rib to the axilla.
4. Brachial a. - from the axilla to the antecubital fossa.
5. Radial a. - from the distal brachial artery to the wrist.
6. Ulnar a. - from the distal brachial artery to the wrist.
7. Palmar arches in hand: deep and superficial.
8. Digital arteries (2 per digit) arise from the palmar arch.

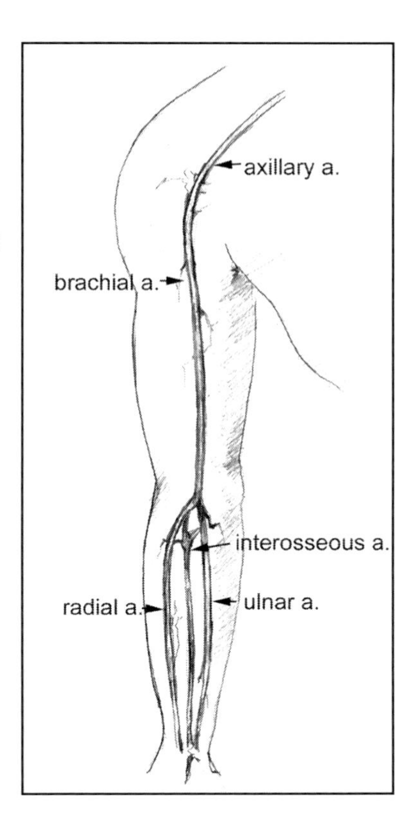

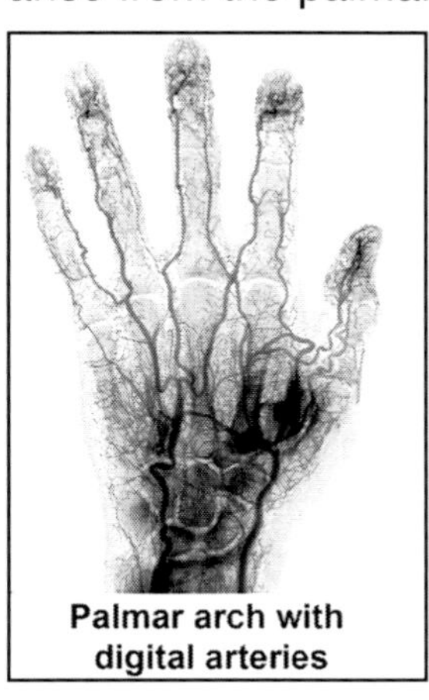
Palmar arch with digital arteries

INDICATIONS

- Arterial insufficiency.
- Weakness in the arm.
- Thoracic Outlet Syndrome (TOS).
- Vasospastic disorder -digit cold sensitivity.
- Digital ischemia.
- Abnormal vertebral artery waveform.
- Pre-operative assessment:
  - ⇒ Hemodialysis access.
  - ⇒ Radial artery harvest for coronary artery bypass graft (CABG).

Contraindications

- No arm pressure measurements should be obtained on an arm with a hemodialysis access. However, PVRs, with reduced inflation pressure, or Doppler waveforms are OK.

DISEASE PROCESSES

Large vessel occlusive disease

- Atherosclerotic obstruction occurs predominately in the subclavian & innominate arteries. The axillary, brachial, radial, & ulnar arteries usually spared.
- Takayasu's and giant cell arteritis are autoimmune disorders that may affect the subclavian arteries.
- Subclavian stenosis/occlusion is diagnosed with comparisons of bilateral brachial systolic pressures: a > 20 mmHg gradient suggests subclavian artery disease on the side with the lower pressure. Also, direct interrogation of the subclavian artery with color duplex is more sensitive than a pressure differential in detecting subclavian artery stenosis.

- Thromboembolism: acute obstruction of the distal arteries caused by emboli from subclavian artery disease, proximal aneurysm, or the heart. The site of obstruction depends on the size of the embolus relative to the size of the artery.

<u>Small vessel occlusive disease- fixed</u>

- Buerger's disease (thromboangiitis obliterans): inflammatory condition of the palmar arch and/or digital arteries leading to small vessel obstruction. Found most often in male smokers.

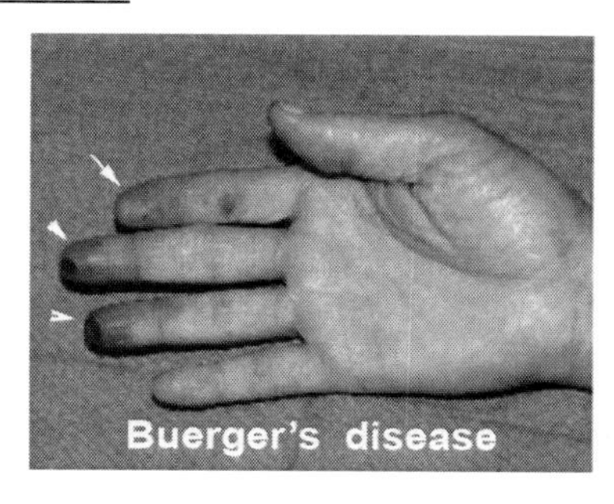

- Thromboemboli: small emboli that occlude the vessels of the hand and digits.

<u>Small vessel vasospastic disorder</u>

- <u>Raynaud's Syndrome</u>: episodic, prolonged digital vasospasm brought about by cold exposure, chemicals (nicotine), emotion, or occupational trauma (vibration injury) to the hands.

  ⇒ Primary Raynaud's Syndrome: a vasospastic disorder without underlying disease. The digital and palmar arteries are without obstruction and perfusion to the digits at rest is normal.

  ⇒ Secondary Raynaud's syndrome: vasospasm associated with an underlying autoimmune disease or connective tissue disease, e.g., scleroderma. The digital/palmar arteries often have <u>fixed obstruction</u>. Even a normal vasoconstrictive response to cold in these patients can cause severe ischemia.

- These were previously differentiated as <u>Raynaud's disease,</u> and <u>Raynaud's phenomenon,</u> respectively.

- Symptoms of the primary syndrome include pallor of digits during vasospasm, followed by cyanosis and rubor upon release of the spasm. The spasm may take 10-30 minutes to release. Small vessel vasospasm occurs normally in response to cold exposure and is triggered by the sympathetic nervous system. In some individuals, however, a sympathetic over-activity occurs that causes the vasospasm to occur with less provocation. Following the vasospastic response, or the removal of the condition that triggered the effect, the spasm does not quit.

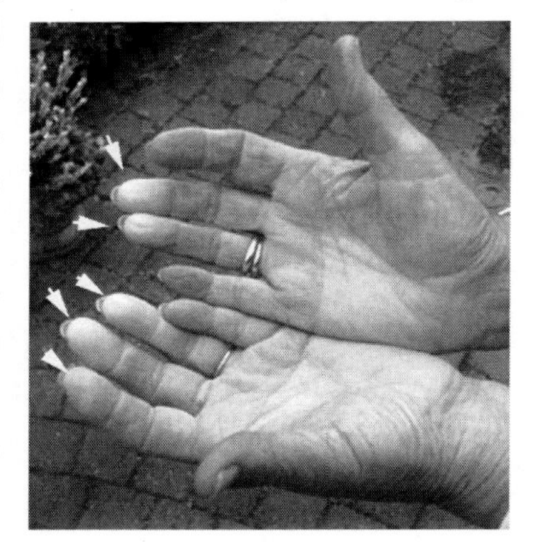

- Typically, the affected area turns white, then blue, then often to bright red.
- Symptoms include numbness and pain.
- Digit vessels may eventually thrombose.

RAYNAUD'S SYNDROME:

- 70-90% of cases occur in females.
- 40% related to connective tissue disorders (scleroderma, lupus, rheumatoid arthritis).
- 40% idiopathic.
- 20% other etiology, frostbite, repetitive vibration injury, etc.

Treatment:

- Cessation of smoking.
- Cold/stress avoidance.
- Calcium channel blockers: Procardia, Nicardipine.

- Sympathetic blocking agents.
- Treat associated disease.
- Cervico-thoracic sympathectomy.
- Micro-revascularization.
- Relocation to warm climate.

THORACIC OUTLET SYNDROME (TOS)

- Intermittent pain, numbness, or weakness of arm(s) related to arm position. Caused by compression of artery or nerve by the anterior scalene muscle, clavicle, rib, or congenital muscular anomalies.
- 95% of TOS is of neurogenic etiology, i.e., compression of the brachial plexus.
- Less than 5% is vascular compression in which the subclavian/axillary artery flow is compromised.
- TOS may cause thrombosis, fibrosis, and aneurysm of the subclavian or axillary arteries.

INDIRECT TEST METHODS

Baseline exam- Rule out arterial occlusive disease

1. Introduce yourself to your patient prior to the test.
2. Obtain a pertinent history of symptoms, including duration, location, and whether persistent or episodic. Note HX of smoking, diabetes, MI, and vascular bypass operations.
3. With the patient in a sitting position, obtain segmental systolic pressures at the arm and the forearm levels, bilaterally.
4. Obtain pulse volume recordings (PVR) from the same sites, or acquire CW Doppler waveform tracings from the axillary, brachial, radial and ulnar arteries.

5. Obtain a PVR, photoplethysmography (PPG) waveform or pressures from both index fingers.

6. If the patient complains of arm pain/numbness/weakness that is position related, perform Thoracic Outlet Test described below.

Tailor subsequent testing for the patient's symptoms.

⇒ Position-related arm pain, numbness or weakness- perform thoracic outlet test.

⇒ Ischemic digits - perform upper extremity and digit physiologic exam.

⇒ Episodic vasospasm- perform baseline digit exam and cold immersion study.

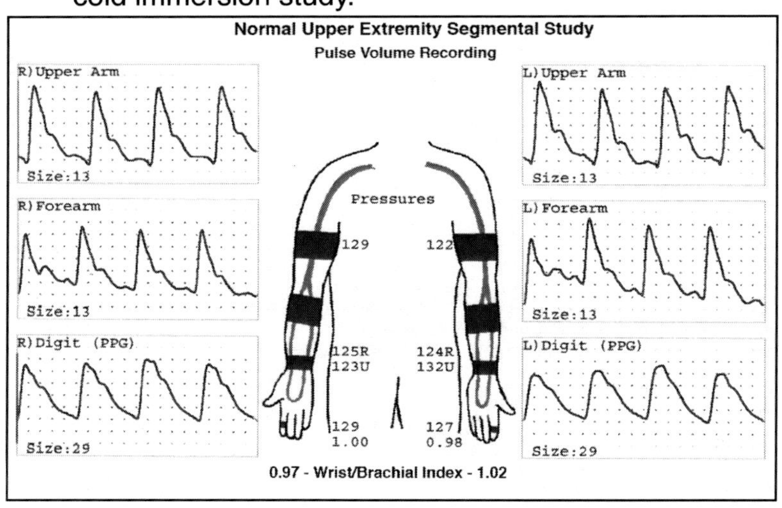

Thoracic Outlet Test Method

- After the baseline study has been performed, obtain a waveform with one following methods to serve as a baseline reference for positional TOS study:
  - a) Photoplethysmography (PPG) on the index fingers.
  - b) Pulse volume recording (PVRs) of the arms.

c) CW-Doppler tracings from the radial or ulnar arteries.

- Next, obtain tracings from both arms either bilaterally, if instrumentation allows, or unilaterally in each of the following arm positions:

  1. Abducted 90 degrees to the torso.
  2. Elevated 180 degrees above the head.
  3. Arm abducted 90 degrees, with elbow bend 90 degrees ("pledge" position). Evaluate with the head turned toward, then away from the hand (modified Adson's maneuver).
  4. Elbows at side and pressed backwards, hands up, shoulders pressed downward and back ("stick-up" position).
  5. Symptomatic position.

MOST IMPORTANT, evaluate in the symptomatic position.

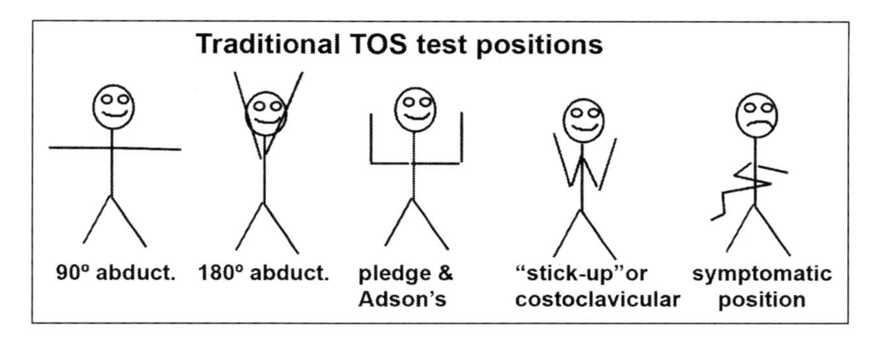

TOS Interpretation

- The amplitude of waveform tracings should remain similar to or larger than baseline tracings in any of the arm positions.
- A significant and sustained decrease in amplitude suggests vascular compression.

- The definitive positive finding is a loss of pulsatility or "flatline" waveform with the patient in a symptomatic condition.
- Often, in a patient with vascular TOS, small changes in arm position can restore or diminish the waveform tracing. Below is a positive TOS study.

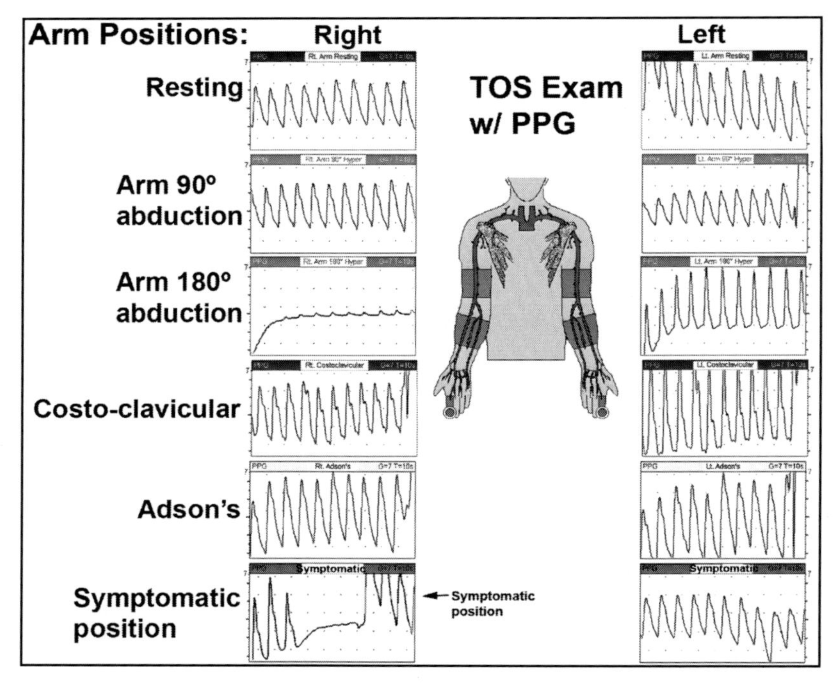

TOS TEST. PPG sensors record perfusion from both index fingers. There is reduced right arm perfusion in the 180° elevated position. This corresponded with the patient's symptomatic position. This is a positive study for right arm vascular TOS.

TOS Pitfalls

In some otherwise normal patients the PPG tracings may go "flatline" when the arm is raised over the head (180°) and if their hand is hyperextended. If this occurs, ask that they relax their fingers, then reassess. If the flat line tracings persist, confirm this positive finding with a CW Doppler held over the radial or ulnar artery in the same arm position. Another false positive result can occur if the Doppler probe slips off the radial or ulnar artery in any arm position. This, of course, would result in a reduced or absent Doppler signal and tracing.

Baseline Physiologic Digital Exam

Using the procedures described below, determine whether digital perfusion is normal or abnormal. If abnormal, determine whether the cause is small vessel fixed obstructive disease, e.g., Buerger's disease, or vasospasm disorder.

Digital exams should be performed in a comfortably warm room to avoid vasoconstriction.

- Evaluate all digits with one of the following methods:

    a) PVRs with digital pressure cuffs.

    b) PPGs obtained distally.

    c) Digit pressures using PPG and digital pressure cuffs.

    d) Duplex imaging of the digits (with a high frequency transducers) is an option if there is evidence for fixed obstruction.

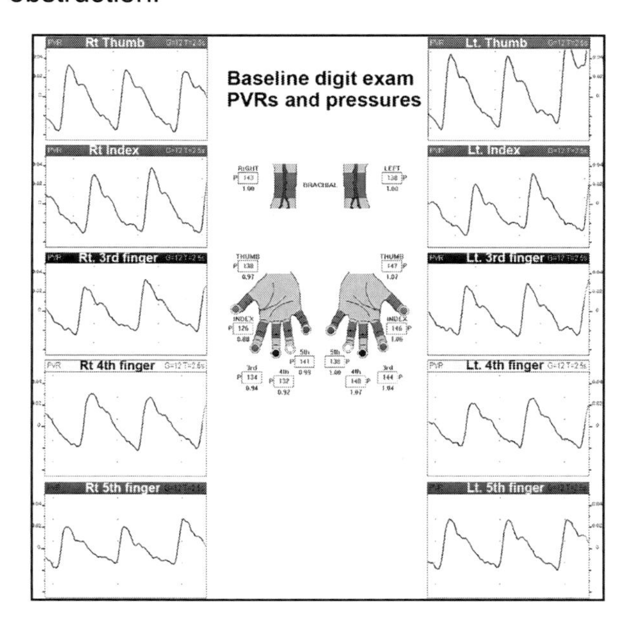

If perfusion is normal or near normal and the patient is symptomatic for Raynaud's Syndrome, perform TEST "A" described below. If digital tracings are abnormal at rest, proceed to TEST "B".

Raynaud's exam

Test "A", Cold Immersion test

⇒ Record pre-submersion PVRs or PPGs on the symptomatic digits.

⇒ Remove the PPG sensors and place the symptomatic hand(s) in a plastic bag. Submerge the hand(s) into a basin of ice water for 1-2 minutes, or less, if the patient is unable to tolerate the discomfort/ pain. This technique keeps the hand dry, and the PVR cuff may be left on. Hands may be immersed without the plastic bag after removing sensors/cuffs, but the hand must be dried and sensors or cuffs reapplied after submersion.

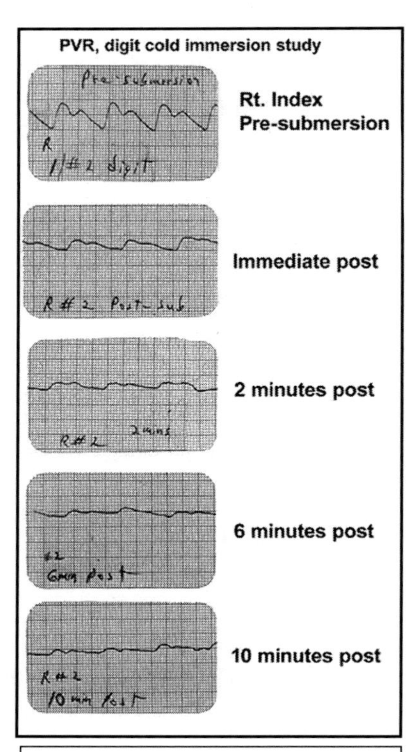

Abnormal cold immersion test of the right index finger; the PVR waveforms are persistently dampened even 10 minutes after cessation of cold stimulation.

⇒ Obtain post submersion tracings on the symptomatic digits using whatever method was used in pre-submersion test.

⇒ Obtain tracings at 2 or 3 minutes intervals thereafter. If PVR amplitude returns to baseline levels within 5 minutes, you may discontinue testing as this represents a normal exam.

⇒ If waveform amplitude remains low, continue recording at 2 minute intervals until 10 minutes has elapsed since the first post-submersion tracing. A persistent decrease in digital waveform amplitude, as compared to baseline pre-submersion tracings, at 10 minutes or longer confirms a vasospastic disorder, or Raynaud's syndrome.

Testing for Raynaud's can also be performed with digit temperature sensors and cold immersion. Infrared temperature sensors or thermistors are used to acquire digital temperatures in a similar sequence to those described above. Failure to return to baseline temperatures within 5 minutes constitutes a positive exam.

Test "B"

If digital PVR or PPG tracings are abnormal at rest, the patient may have occlusive disease, secondary Raynaud's, Buerger's etc., or they may be experiencing vasoconstriction or vasospasm.

⇒ Ensure that the exam room is warm.

⇒ Wrap the affected hand in a heating pad and warm for 5 minutes.

⇒ Repeat digit PVRs or PPGs following re-warming. If waveform amplitudes remain abnormal, small vessel occlusive disease should be suspected. If amplitudes become normal following warming, a vasospasm/ vasoconstrictive condition exists.

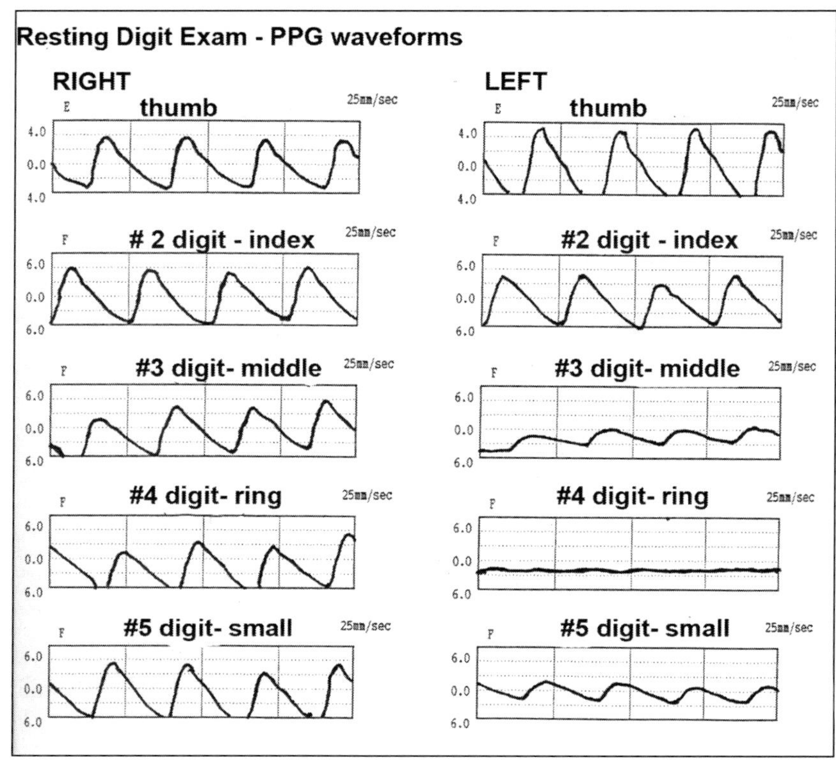

A 62-year-old male presented with numbness and ischemic changed on his left 4th and 5th digits distally. No history of smoking or prior cold sensitivity. The arm physiologic study was normal. PPG waveforms were abnormal in the left 3rd, 4th, and 5th digits indicating reduced perfusion. Both hands were warmed in a heating blanket for 10 minutes and digits were retested.

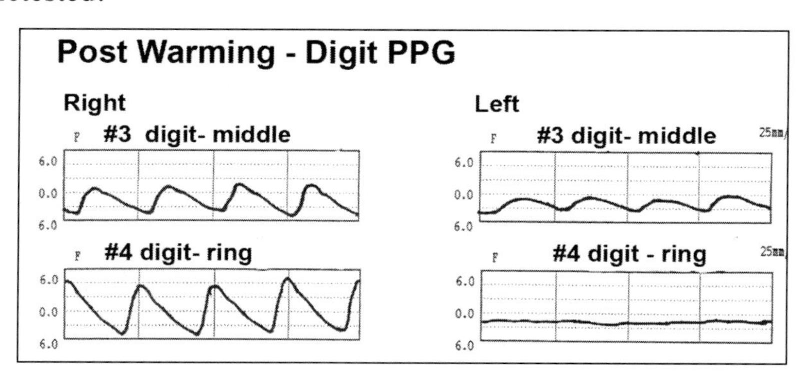

Following rewarming there was no improvement in perfusion to the affected digits on the left hand. This finding suggested fixed occlusive disease, as opposed to vasospasm. The digits were imaged with a high frequency intraoperative ultrasound transducer and digital artery occlusion was found in the involved fingers. Ultrasound scan of the left subclavian artery for aneurysm was negative. Due to a suspicion of thromboemboli as the cause of the occlusions, the patient was scheduled for an echocardiogram. The results were unavailable.

ALLEN TEST FOR PALMAR ARCH PATENCY

This exam is essential prior to radial artery harvest for coronary artery bypass surgery and prior to ipsilateral hemodialysis fistula or graft implantation. If the radial artery is removed in a patient that is "radial dominant", and if the palmar arch is not intact, severe ischemia may result in the fingers and hand. Radial artery "steal" phenomenon is not uncommon in Brescia-Cimino dialysis fistulas. The "steal" condition is usually benign as long as the palmar arch is complete.

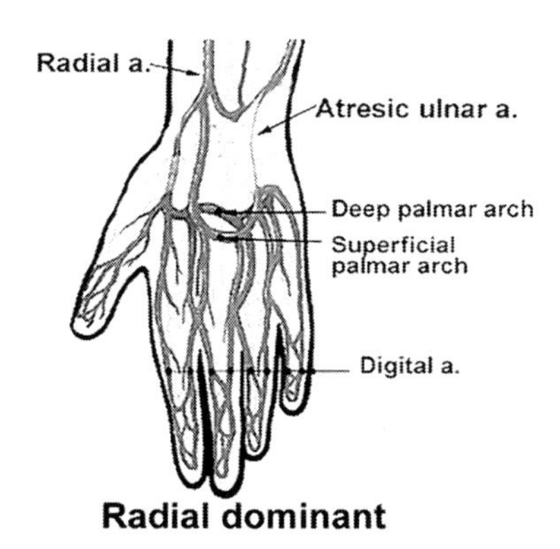

Radial dominant

The Allen test may be performed manually without instrumentation, or with monitoring devices (PPG, PVR or digit pressures) on the thumb or index finger and the little finger. A standard resting digit exam should be performed on all fingers prior to the Allen test.

Manual Exam

1. Occlude the patient's radial and ulnar arteries with your thumbs, and have the patient squeeze their fist 3-4 times to exsanguinate (empty) the blood out of the hand.
2. Release only one of the arteries and observe whether the palm becomes pink (perfused) across the entire hand and digits.
3. Repeat arterial compression and hand squeeze, then release the other artery and observe normal or abnormal cutaneous filling.
4. Absence of capillary refilling suggests an occluded palmar arch or radial/ulnar dominance.

PPG testing for Palmar Arch Patency

The test for Palmar arch patency can be performed with an Allen test but it's best performed with physiologic testing devices.

- Photoplethysmography (PPG) sensors are placed on the thumb or index finger and the 5th digit (if a 2 channel system is available).
- The PPG scale or gain controls are adjusted to establish similar amplitudes.
- Use a slow sweep speed and if possible, monitor both digits simultaneously.
- Compress and hold both the radial artery (RA) and ulnar arteries with your thumbs simultaneously, and observe changes in the PPG trace of the two digits. The tracings should be "flat line" during compression. This ensures that your compressions are adequate. If the waveforms are not obliterated, reposition your thumbs over the RA and UA, and try again, see figure A below.

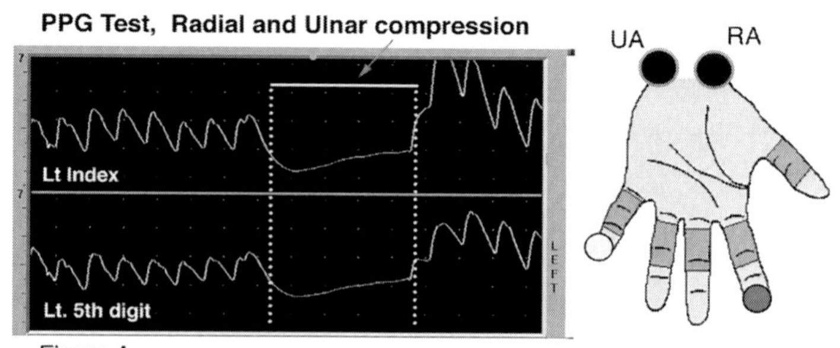

Figure A.

- Repeat the test, compressing the radial artery; record the waveforms. Repeat the test with ulnar compression. A normal response is indicated by little or no decrease in PPG waveform amplitude, see figure B below.

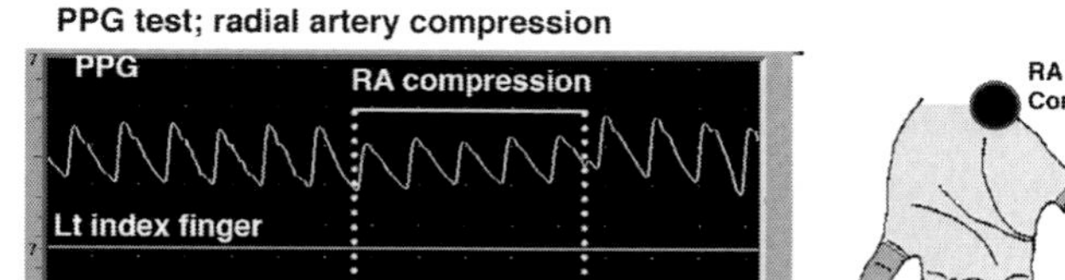

Figure B.

- If all the PPG waveforms drop to flat-line (as in Figure A above) or nearly flat-line with radial artery compression, the patient is <u>radial dominate</u> and a radial artery harvest is contraindicated. This indicates that the ulnar artery cannot perfuse the hand if you "take the radial out of the circuit".

- If the PPGs go flat line with ulnar artery compression, the patient is <u>ulnar dominate</u>. The radial artery can be harvested if there are no other complications.

- Digital pressures are useful when there is a partial decrease in perfusion during radial artery compression with PPG monitoring. This provides a quantitative measure of digit perfusion. It is not necessary (or possible) to attempt to obtain a digit pressure on a finger with a flatline PPG tracing!

Digit pressures with RA compression

- Obtain thumb or index digit pressures at rest.
- While compressing the radial artery, re-obtain digit pressure and compare to resting value.
- In the image below, the patient has decreased PPG amplitude with RA compression indicating a partially intact palmar arch. Thumb pressure was obtained at rest (147 mmHg), and during radial compression (79 mmHg). This pressure should be sufficient to maintain digit viability if the radial artery is removed.

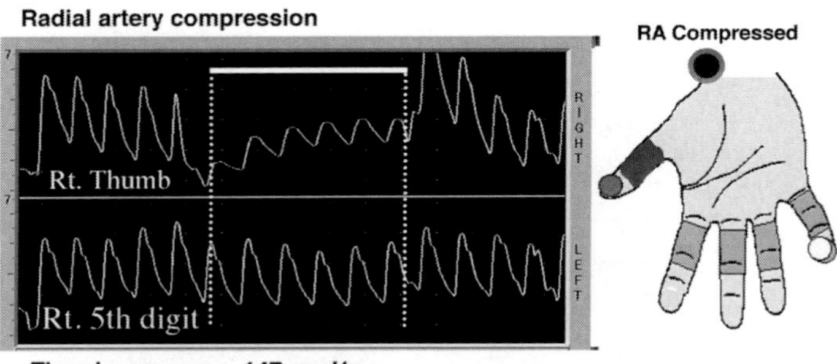

Thumb pressure = 147 mmHg
Thumb pressure with RA compression = 79 mmHg

CHAPTER 7: REIMBURSEMENT

This chapter will provide basic information on CPT codes and reimbursement that is current to September 2013. Because Medicare Part B guidelines and regulations may change at any time in the future, updates (if any) to the content of this chapter will be provided on our website at www.summerpublishing.com.

THE INFORMATION PROVIDED WITH THIS CHAPTER IS GENERAL REIMBURSEMENT INFORMATION ONLY; IT IS NOT LEGAL ADVICE, NOR IS IT ADVICE ABOUT HOW TO CODE, COMPLETE OR SUBMIT ANY PARTICULAR CLAIM FOR PAYMENT.

CPT AND ICD-9-CM OVERVIEW

Current Procedural Terminology (CPT®) codes are created and controlled by the American Medical Association and are the basis for reimbursement by Medicare, Medicaid and by insurance companies.

The Healthcare Common Procedure Coding System (HCPCS) are codes based on the CPT to provide standardized coding when healthcare is delivered.

CPT codes describe medical, surgical, and diagnostic services and are designed to communicate uniform information about medical services and procedures among physicians, coders, patients, accreditation organizations, and payers for administrative, financial, and analytical purposes. from Wikipedia.

The International Classification of Diseases, Ninth Revision (ICD-9) is the classification used to code and classify mortality data from death certificates. It's often used interchangeably with ICD-9-CM. ICD-9-CM (Clinical Modification) is a system for assigning codes to diagnoses and procedures associated with hospital utilization in the United States.

An ICD-9-CM code must accompany a CPT code when a claim is submitted for reimbursement, and the ICD-9-CM code must match the CPT code. For example, if an arterial CPT code is submitted and the ICD-9-CM code is for a venous symptom, the claim will most likely be rejected.

In 2014 the ICD codes will change to the 10th version (ICD-10-CM).

There are national mandates established by Centers for Medicare and Medicaid Services (CMS) that apply to all Medicare Part B service provider. There are also Local Coverage Determinations (LCD) rules that vary by region or state.

Two of the national coverage determination worth mentioning:

1. Medicare will not reimburse for a venous exam and an arterial exam performed on the same patient, on the same day. There is an exception; if you can provide clearly documented different and divergent symptoms, and you can demonstrate medical necessity. (This applies more to vascular ultrasound than to physiologic testing).
2. Medical necessity for the physiologic testing, as in all procedures, must be established and clearly documented.

ABI NOMENCLATURE

One of the national mandates specifies that the acquisition of the ABI is considered part of the physical examination of the patient, and it is not reimbursable. The term ABI means ankle to brachial index, but sometimes the "phrase" is used (incorrectly) to mean ABI with ankle waveforms, either Doppler or PVR waveforms. The ABI with waveforms is technically a "limited bilateral noninvasive physiologic studies of lower extremity arteries" and it is reimbursable.

WHO CAN PERFORM THE EXAMS?

Regional Medicare contractors will either "recommend" a level of training and credentialing, or they will <u>mandate</u> it. Please check with your regional Medicare contractor for the regulations on noninvasive vascular testing. The Intersocietal Accreditation Commission (IAC) is a good source for current reimbursement information by State or contractor.

(http://intersocietal.org/vascular/main/payment_policies.htm)

The following is quoted from the LCDs for Colorado; the Medicare contractor is Novitas Solutions.[1]

"The accuracy of noninvasive vascular studies depends on the knowledge, skill and experience of the technologist and physician performing and interpreting the study. Consequently, the providers of interpretations must be capable of demonstrating documented training and experience and maintain documentation for post-payment audit. A vascular diagnostic study may be personally performed by a physician or a technologist."

"All noninvasive vascular diagnostic studies performed by a technologist must be either (1) performed by, or under the direct supervision of, a technologist who has demonstrated competency by being credentialed in vascular technology, (2) performed under the direct supervision of a physician capable of demonstrating training and experience specific to the study performed, 3) performed in a facility accredited by the Intersocietal Commission for the Accreditation of Vascular Laboratories (ICAVL) or the Non-Invasive Vascular Ultrasound Accreditation of the American College of Radiology (ACR). "

"Examples of appropriate personnel certification include the Registered Vascular Technologist (RVT) credential and the Registered Vascular Specialist (RVS) credential in Vascular Technology."

Some contractors include American Registry of Radiologic Technologists with Vascular Sonography (VS).

Summary: you can perform testing if:

1) you are credentialed as an RVT, RVS, or VS.
2) your lab is accredited by IAC (formerly ICAVL), or ACR.
3) you are under the direct supervision of an RVT, RVS, VS.
4) you are a physician who is competent in diagnostic vascular studies.
5) the interpreting physician must demonstrate documented training and experience in noninvasive vascular interpretation (the ARDMS RPVI credential would fulfill this requirement).

Some Medicare contractors indicate the exam can be performed by or under the direct supervision of a physician (who is competent in diagnostic vascular studies). Others might recommend, but not require, the standards listed above.

Direct supervision is defined by CMS as:

"Direct supervision in the office setting means the physician (or the credentialed technologist) must be present in the office suite and be immediately available (and "interruptible") to furnish assistance and direction throughout the performance of the procedure. It does not mean that the physician must be present in the room when the procedure is performed."

There are 3 CPT codes used for non-invasive peripheral arterial studies. Codes cannot be used in tandem on the same patient; only one code should be applied. The CPT codes define minimum requirements for testing.

CPT CODES

93922

Limited, bilateral noninvasive physiologic studies of upper or lower extremity arteries, (e.g., for lower extremity: ankle /brachial indices at distal posterior tibial and anterior tibial/dorsalis pedis arteries plus bi-directional Doppler waveform recording and analysis at 1-2 levels, or ankle /brachial indices at distal posterior tibial and anterior tibial/ dorsalis pedis arteries plus volume plethysmography at 1-2 levels, or ankle /brachial indices at distal posterior tibial and anterior tibial/ dorsalis pedis arteries with transcutaneous oxygen tension ($TCPO_2$) measurements at 1-2 levels.

93922 Analysis: perform one of these options:

1) Obtain ABIs from the arms and distal posterior tibial and dorsalis pedis arteries. Acquire pulse volume recording (PVRs) from ankles bilaterally,

or

2) Obtain ABIs from arms and the distal posterior tibial and dorsalis pedis arteries. Acquire bidirectional CW Doppler waveforms from both PTA and DPA bilaterally.

or

3) Obtain ABIs from the distal posterior tibial and dorsalis pedis arteries. Perform $TCPO_2$ at 1-2 levels (this is an uncommon test used to determine wound healing and amputation levels).

93923

Complete, bilateral noninvasive physiologic studies of upper or lower extremity arteries at 3 or more levels, (e.g., for lower extremity: ankle /brachial indices at distal posterior tibial and anterior tibial/ dorsalis pedis arteries plus segmental blood pressure measurements with bidirectional Doppler waveform recording and analysis, at 3 or more levels, or ankle /brachial indices at distal posterior tibial and anterior tibial/dorsalis pedis arteries plus volume plethysmography at 3 or more levels, or ankle /brachial indices at distal posterior tibial and anterior tibial/dorsalis pedis arteries plus segmental transcutaneous oxygen tension measurements at 3 or more levels, or single level study with provocative functional maneuvers (e.g., measurements with postural provocative tests (toe raises), or measurements with reactive hyperemia).

93923 Analysis: perform one of these options:

1) Obtain ABIs from the PTA and the DPA. Record segmental **PVRs** at the ankle, calf and thigh, bilaterally. Optionally, obtain PVRs from metatarsals and great toes. *Note, segmental pressures (from calf and thigh sites) are optional and not required when segmental PVRs are performed.*

or

2) Obtain ABIs from the PTA and DPA arteries. Obtain blood pressure measurements from the calf, and upper thigh levels (the addition of a lower thigh pressure is optional, and depends on your protocol). Record **CW Doppler waveforms** from the PTA, DPA, Popliteal, SFA and CFA bilaterally.

or

3) Obtain ABIs from the PTA and DPA arteries, plus segmental transcutaneous oxygen tension measurements at three or more level(s).

or

4) Obtain a single level study (see 93922), include provocative functional maneuvers (example, measurements with postural provocative tests, toe raise/heel lifts, or measurements with reactive hyperemia, *Ouch!*).

93924

Noninvasive physiologic studies of lower extremity arteries, at rest and following treadmill stress testing, (i.e., bidirectional Doppler waveform or volume plethysmography recording and analysis at rest with ankle/brachial indices immediately after and at timed intervals following performance of a standardized protocol on a motorized treadmill plus recording of time of onset of claudication or other symptoms, maximal walking time, and time to recovery) complete bilateral study.

93924 Analysis

93924 defines the methods used in 93922, or 93923 to include treadmill stress testing. The description is unclear as to whether a limited study or a complete bilateral resting study is required prior to exercise.

After the resting study is completed, the patient is exercised on a treadmill for a standard walking time, or until they cannot continue. Time of onset of symptoms should be recorded, as well as duration of walking time, treadmill speed and elevation.

ABIs should be obtained as soon as possible following exercise from either the PTA or DPA; use whichever vessel had the higher pressure in the resting study. Perform ABIs at 1-3 minute intervals until the ankle pressures return to baseline (resting) levels. Record the "recovery time".

Toe raises (with post-exercise pressures) or other provocative maneuvers do not qualify for the 93924 code, only treadmill exercise. If toe raises are performed in either a limited or a complete bilateral physiologic study, the 93923 code should be used.

Other reimbursement notes:

To report a unilateral (one side only) study; if three or more levels are measured on one limb use code 93922, if only one or two levels are measured use code 93922 with modifier 52 and provide a reason why it was unilateral. (i.e., Amputation, cellulitis, infectious disease, etc.).

The global charge includes both the professional (26) and the technical components (TC) of the service. The professional component is generally paid based on the Medicare physician fee schedule, but for Category III CPT codes, local Medicare contractors determine the payment rate.

Some Medicare contractors allow reimbursement for color duplex imaging (92925) on the same day, if the physiologic test was positive.

ICD-9-CM; ICD-10-CM

ICD-9-CM codes must be used in conjunction with a CPT code. The following is a list of commonly used ICD-9-CM codes linked with 92922, 93923, and 93924 for peripheral arterial disease. The 400 series is ICD-9-CM, the codes in parentheses are the new ICD-10-CM for 2014.

250.70 (E11.51)	Diabetes with peripheral circulatory disorders-type II, not stated as controlled.
440.0 (I70.0)	Atherosclerosis of aorta
440.21 (I70.219)	Atherosclerosis of the extremities with intermittent claudication
440.22 (I70.229)	Atherosclerosis of the extremities with rest pain
440.23 (I70.25)	Atherosclerosis of the extremities with ulceration
440.24 (I70.269)	Atherosclerosis of the extremities with gangrene
440.29 (I70.299)	Atherosclerosis of the extremities, other
442.0 (I72.1)	Aneurysm of artery of upper extremity
442.3 (I72.4)	Aneurysm of artery of lower extremity
443.0 – 443.9	Other peripheral vascular diseases
443.0 (I73.00)	Raynaud's syndrome, without gangrene
443.1 (I73.1)	Thromboangiitis obliterans (Buerger's disease)
443.9 (I73.9)	Peripheral vascular disease unspecified
444.21 (I74.2)	Arterial embolism and thrombosis of arteries of upper extremities
444.22 (I74.3)	Arterial embolism and thrombosis of lower extremities.

References

1. Novitas Solutions. https://www.novitas-solutions.com/policy/mac-ab/l30827-r5.html

CME CREDIT INFORMATION

- Six (6) continuing medical education (CME) credits have been approved for this self-study program through the Society for Vascular Ultrasound.
- *The CME post-test application and test can be found on our website:* **www.Summerpublishing.com.**
- SVU CME credits may be applied towards the CME requirements of the ARDMS, the ARRT, CCI, and CARDUP, as well as ICAVL and ACR accreditation organizations. Please note that these are NOT AMA category 1 credits (often required for physician medical director accreditation).
- CME credits have been approved through 2/17/2016. Please check our website for updated CME information and renewal.
- Select the CME Information page, and download the PDF document. You must have Adobe Reader software to read the PDF document. A free download of the Reader software is available at www.adobe.com.
- Fax the completed application, completed test answer sheet, and evaluation form, along with credit card number to: 866-519-0674. The fax line is secure. Alternatively, the completed application, with check or credit card number, can be mailed to:

Summer Publishing
CME Administrator
4572 Christensen Circle
Littleton, CO 80123-6500

There is no need to send the application via special delivery, or signature required service.

- The test consists of 40 multiple choice questions.

- Additional lab personnel may take the exam after studying the book. Download a different test version from the website. ONLY ONE TEST IS REQUIRED PER PERSON.

Course Objectives: Upon completion of reading and studying " A Pocket Guide to Physiologic Arterial Testing", the participant should be able to:

1. Describe basic Doppler fundamentals as they apply to physiologic arterial testing.
2. Define upper and lower arterial anatomy.
3. Discuss normal arterial hemodynamics and how flow patterns are altered by disease.
4. List diagnostic criteria for lower arterial physiologic diagnostic exams.
5. Describe and understand instrumentation used in physiologic testing of the extremities for peripheral arterial disease (PAD).
6. Utilize indirect testing methods to detect subclavian artery stenosis and thoracic outlet syndrome.
7. Describe test methods to detect digit diseases including Raynaud's Syndrome and Buerger's Disease.
8. Describe test protocols as they relate to CPT code guidelines.
9. Interpret physiologic arterial exams for various disease levels based on case study reviews.
10. Identify and apply ICD-9 and new ICD-10 codes for improved reimbursement success.

BOOK CODE 72747